Practical Obstetric Hematology

Practical Obstetric Hematology

Peter Clark BSc MD FRCP FRCPath
Consultant Haematologist
Department of Transfusion Medicine, Ninewells Hospital
and Medical School, Dundee, UK

Ian A Greer MD FRCP FRCOG MFFP
Regius Professor of Obstetrics & Gynaecology
University of Glasgow,
Glasgow, UK

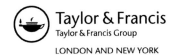

Taylor & Francis
Taylor & Francis Group

LONDON AND NEW YORK

© 2006 Taylor & Francis, an imprint of the Taylor & Francis Group
Taylor & Francis Group is the Academic Division of T&F Informa plc

First published in the United Kingdom in 2006 by Taylor & Francis, an imprint of the Taylor & Francis Group, 2 Park Square, Milton Park, Abingdon, Oxon OX14 4RN

Tel.:   +44 (0)20 7017 6000
Fax.:   +44 (0)20 7017 6699
E-mail: info.medicine@tandf.co.uk
Website: www.tandf.co.uk/medicine

Although every effort has been made to ensure that drug doses and other information are presented accurately in this publication, the ultimate responsibility rests with the prescribing physician. Neither the publishers nor the authors can be held responsible for errors or for any consequences arising from the use of information contained herein. For detailed prescribing information or instructions on the use of any product or procedure discussed herein, please consult the prescribing information or instructional material issued by the manufacturer.

A CIP record for this book is available from the British Library.

Library of Congress Cataloging-in-Publication Data

Data available on application

ISBN 1-84214-262-3
ISBN 978-1-84214-262-2

Distributed in North and South America by

Taylor & Francis
2000 NW Corporate Blvd
Boca Raton, FL 33431, USA

Within Continental USA
Tel: 800 272 7737; Fax: 800 374 3401
Outside Continental USA
Tel: 561 994 0555; Fax: 561 361 6018
E-mail:

Distributed in the rest of the world by
Thomson Publishing Services
Cheriton House
North Way
Andover, Hampshire SP10 5BE, UK
Tel: +44 (0)1264 332424
E-mail: salesorder.tandf@thomsonpublishingservices.co.uk

Composition by Tek-Art, Croydon, Surrey

Printed and bound in the UK by TJ International, Padstow, Cornwall

Contents

Preface

In the last 10 years there has been a rapid expansion in the clinical interaction between hematologists and obstetricians. As a result there is an increasing challenge to hematologists, obstetricians and midwifery staff to understand and manage the clinical manifestations of a number of rapidly developing areas of hemato-obstetric science.

This book is intended to serve practitioners involved in the management of pregnancy, from trainees in obstetrics, hematology and vascular medicine to general practitioners involved in the day-to-day management of maternity care, as well as midwifery staff and specialists in hematology, obstetrics and vascular medicine. The book is designed to assist the reader to diagnose and treat these conditions, but also provides the reader with a user-friendly, but authoritative, source of information on the pathophysiology of hemato-obstetric problems that incorporates the best practice contained within internationally accepted guidelines of obstetric and hematological care.

The book is intended to assist the reader rapidly assimilate the essential aspects of the pathophysiology of these complex disorders and provide an aide memoir to the management of these conditions. As well as a guide to the pitfalls associated with investigation and treatment, each chapter has a similar format and employs extensive use of tables and figures.

The first chapter covers the physiological changes in hematological indices caused by normal pregnancy. The second provides a succinct review of the basic science of transfusion medicine and appropriate blood component usage as it relates to obstetric practice. The subsequent chapters deal with the impact, diagnosis and management of adverse transfusion events, hemolytic disease of the newborn, anemia, malignant hematology, bleeding disorders, antithrombotic therapy, thrombophilia, thrombotic disorders and red cell disorders in pregnancy.

To assist the reader, each of these chapters conforms to a similar style that includes: pathophysiology; presentation; differential diagnosis; diagnostic tests; diagnostic difficulties; maternal complications, fetal complications; and potential management complications. Each chapter also includes tables summarizing the key points in diagnosis and management, as well as information on the likely impact of new therapies and a preview of the developing issues relating to each condition.

Glossary

ACCP	American College of Chest Physicians
ACE	Angiotensin-converting enzyme
ADAMTS	A disintegrin and metalloproteinase with thrombospondin domains
ADP	Adenosine diphosphate
AF	Atrial fibrillation
AFLP	Acute fatty liver of pregnancy
AIHA	Autoimmune hemolytic anemia
AIN	Autoimmune neutropenia
AIP	Acute intermittent porphyria
AML	Acute myeloid leukemia
APAS	Antiphospholipid antibody syndrome
aPC	Activated protein C
aPCR	Activated protein C resistance
APS	Antiphospholipid syndrome
APTT	Activated partial thromboplastin time
Art T	Arterial thrombosis
AST	Aspartate Transaminase
AT	Antithrombin
ATP	Adenosine triphosphate
BMI	Body mass index
CD	Cluster of differentiation
CEP	Congenital erythropoietic porphyria
CI	Confidence interval
CIAO	Cerebral ischemia of arterial origin
CMV	Cytomegalovirus
CNS	Central nervous system
CT	Computerized tomography
CTG	Cardiotocography
CVP	Chorionic villus sampling
DDAVP	Demopressin analog
DIC	Disseminated intravascular coagulation

2,3-DPG	2,3-diphosphoglycerate
dRVVT	Dilute Russell viper venom test
DVT	Deep vein thrombosis
ECG	Electrocardiogram
EDTA	Ethylenediaminetetraacetic acid
ELISA	Enzyme-linked immunosorbent assay
EPCR	Endothelial protein C receptor
Epo	Erythropoietin
EPP	Erythropoietic protoporphyria
ET	Essential thrombocythemia
F	Factor
FBC	Full blood count
FDP	Fibrin degradation products
FFP	Fresh frozen plasma
FMH	Feto-maternal hemorrhage
FPA	Fibrinopeptide A
G6PDH	Glucose-6-phosphate dehydrogenase
G-CSF	Granulocyte colony-stimulating factor
GI	Gastrointestinal
GPI	Glycophosphatidylinositol
GVHD	Graph-versus host disease
Hb	Hemoglobin
HCY	Homocysteine
HDN	Hemolytic disease of the newborn
HELLP	Hemolysis, elevated liver enzymes, and low platelets
HHV	Human herpes virus
HIT	Heparin-induce thrombocytopenia
HITTS	HIT thrombosis syndrome
HLA	Human leukocyte antigen
HPA	Human platelet antigen
HPFH	Hereditary persistence of fetal hemoglobin
HPLC	High-performance liquid chromatography
HTLV	Human T-cell leukemia/lymphoma virus
HUS	Hemolytic uremic syndrome
ICH	Intracerebral hemorrhage

IDA	Iron deficiency anemia
IgG	Immunoglobulin
INR	International normalized ratio
ISI	International sensitivity index
ITP	Immune thrombocytopenia/idiopathic thrombocytopenic purpura
IUGR	Intrauterine growth restriction
IVIgG	Intravenous human normal IgG
LDH	Lactate dehydrogenase
LDL	Low-density lipoprotein
LFT	Liver function test
LMWH	Low-molecular-weight heparin
MAHA	Microangiopathic hemolytic anemia
MB	Methylene blue
MCH	Mean corpuscular (red cell) hemoglobin
MCV	Mean corpuscular (red cell) volume
MMA	Methylmalonic acid
MRI	Magnetic resonance imaging
MTHFR	Methylene tetrahydrofolate reductase
MTP	Mitochondrial trifunctional protein
NAD	Nicotinamide adenine dinucleotide
NADH	Reduced form of NAD
NADP	Nicotinamide adenine dinucleotide phosphate
NADPH	Reduced form of NADP
NAIT	Neonatal alloimmune thrombocytopenia
NHL	Non-Hodgkin's lymphoma
NNA	Normochromic normocytic anemia
NSAID	Non-steroidal anti-inflammatory drug
nvCJD	New variant Creutzfeldt-Jakob disease
PA	Pernicious anemia
PAI	Plasminogen activator inhibitor
PCR	Polymerase chain reaction
PCT	Porphyria cutanea tarda
PCV	Packed cell volume
PET	Pre-eclampsia
PF	Platelet factor

PMH	Past medical history
PNH	Paroxysmal nocturnal hemoglobinuria
PMN	Polymorphonuclear cell
PPH	Post partum hemorrhage
PT	Prothrombin time
PTE	Pulmonary thromboembolism
PTP	Post-transfusional purpura
PTT	Partial thromboplastin time
RA	Rheumatoid arthritis
rbc	Red blood cell
RFLP	Restriction Fragment Length Polymorphism
rFVIIa	Recombinant FVIIIa
RiCoF	Ristocetin cofactor
rtPA	Recombinant tissue plasminogen activator
SD-FFP	Solvent detergent-treated FFP
SLE	Systemic lupus erythematosis
stfR	Serum transferrin receptor
TAFI	Thrombin-activatable fibrinolysis inhibitor
TA-GVHD	Transfusion-associated graft versus host disease
TAT	Thrombin–antithrombin complex
TCT	Thrombin clotting time
TF	Tissue factor
TFPI	Tissue factor pathway inhibitor
tfR	Transferrin receptor
TIBC	Total iron-binding capacity
tPA	Tissue plasminogen activator
TRALI	Transfusion-related acute lung injury
TT	Thrombin clotting time
TTP	Thrombotic thrombocytopenic purpura
UFH	Unfractionated heparin
U/Q	Ventilation/Perfusion
VTE	Venous thromboembolism
vWD	von Willebrand's disease
vWF	von Willebrand Factor

CHAPTER 1

Hematology measurements in pregnancy

Pregnancy results in significant changes in metabolism, fluid balance, organ function and circulation, which are driven, in part, by estrogen and the presence of the feto-placental unit. These dramatic changes influence a wide variety of hematological parameters. A knowledge of these changes is essential when interpreting the results of hematological investigations to diagnose, or monitor, illness in pregnancy.

Blood count

The maternal plasma volume begins to increase from around 6 weeks gestation, but this is not accompanied by an immediate increase in red cell mass. The effect of this is a dilutional anemia, which may be evident from the 7–8th week of gestation. Although the mechanism of this increase in blood volume is not fully understood, it may be more marked in multiple pregnancies and occurs even when iron stores are poor. The physiological purpose of this change may be to reduce maternal blood viscosity, and improve delivery of oxygen and nutrients to the fetus. The increase in plasma volume may reach 140% of non-pregnant values and usually becomes maximal in the late second trimester. By this stage in pregnancy, a 15–25% increase in red cell mass, driven by an increase in maternal erythropoietin production, will also be present. These changes should not, however, reduce the hemoglobin to <11g/dl in the first trimester or <10g/dl in the second and third trimesters, and should result in a normochromic, normocytic red blood cell pattern on the blood film. This 'physiological anemia' of pregnancy does not worsen during the third trimester, which may reflect a reduction in maternal plasma volume and a stable red cell mass. Consequently, a relative increase in hemoglobin and hematocrit may be observed in the late third trimester.

With normal pregnancy there may also be a rise in the mean corpuscular volume (MCV), and a normal MCV does not, therefore, exclude iron deficiency. Similarly, a modestly elevated MCV does not diagnose folate (or vitamin B_{12}) deficiency in pregnancy (Table 1.1).

Table 1.1 – Blood count and hematinics in normal pregnancy

Parameter	Change in pregnancy
Hemoglobin	Falls, but >11g/dl in the first trimester and >10g/dl in the second and third trimesters
Mean corpuscular volume (MCV)	No change, rise or fall all possible
Platelets	$>80 \times 10^9/l$
Neutrophils	Variable rise (earlier forms seen)
Vitamin B_{12}	<50% fall with increasing gestation
Serum folate	<30% fall with increasing gestation
Red cell folate	<20% rise, or no change with increasing gestation
Homocysteine	No change, or fall
Vitamin B_6	<20% fall with increasing gestation
Fe	Variable fall with increasing gestation
Ferritin	Variable fall; can be reduced to near non-pregnant iron-deficient ranges
Total iron-binding capacity (TIBC)	Variable rise with increasing gestation
Transferrin receptors (tfR)	Increase after 20/40 weeks gestation

Towards the end of pregnancy at least 5% of women have a platelet count below the usual non-pregnant reference range ($150-400 \times 10^9/l$). The majority of these lie above $80-100 \times 10^9/l$, although platelet counts as low as $50 \times 10^9/l$ without significant disease have been reported. This gestational thrombocytopenia is caused by a combination of hemodilution and an increase in platelet activation and clearance, which is partly compensated for by an increase in platelet production and an increased proportion of younger, larger, platelets. The evidence that an increase in platelet activation and clearance occurs includes: an increase in mean platelet volume; an increase in the plasma concentration of the platelet-specific protein β-thromboglobulin in the second and third trimesters; and an increase in the metabolites of the prostanoid thromboxane A_2 (which is released following platelet activation, and which itself is a potent stimulus to platelet activation and aggregation). Following delivery, the platelet count increases in reaction to, and in compensation for, platelet consumption.

Normal pregnancy is associated with a rise in total white blood cell count. This usually results in a mild neutrophilia ($<15 \times 10^9/l$), but earlier granulocyte forms, such as myelocytes and band forms, and a white count of $15-20 \times 10^9/l$ is not uncommon even in normal pregnancies. The presence of these more 'primitive' white cells may result in such samples being 'flagged' as abnormal in automated white cell analyzers. Furthermore, the use of corticosteroids to assist in lung maturation may result in maternal neutrophilia, and the process of delivery itself will often precipitate a brisk leukocytosis.

Hematinic assessment

Normal pregnancy is associated with a progressive fall in serum iron levels and an increase in serum total iron-binding capacity (TIBC: see Chapter 3). The TIBC reflects the amount of the iron transport protein (transferrin) that is saturated with iron; the level of TIBC fluctuates widely and is also influenced by recent iron ingestion. A fall in serum ferritin levels also occurs in normal pregnancy, although very low ferritin levels (<12ug/l) will still reliably indicate iron deficiency. A number of newer tests of iron deficiency have been evaluated out-with pregnancy. These include the plasma level of free transferrin receptors (tfR) and the plasma level of free protoporphyrin. In the latter case, iron deficiency leads to a reduction in the incorporation of iron into the prophyrin ring that forms the heme moiety of hemoglobin. The level of the 'unused' protoporphyrin is therefore a measure of deficiency. However, an increase in free protoporphyrin occurs in normal pregnancy. The tfR is a transmembrane protein that mediates delivery of iron to the developing erythroblast and is shed from the maturing red cell. The serum tfr (stfR) level relates to the degree of iron deficiency and increasing values precede changes in red cell morphology. stfR has been used successfully to discriminate iron deficiency from the anemia of chronic disease, as it does not increase in response to inflammation. However, stfR levels have been shown to increase with gestation, returning to non-pregnant values 3 months postpartum. Although this could relate to undiagnosed iron deficiency, it seems more likely to be due to an increase in maternal erythropoiesis.

Vitamin B_{12} levels may fall by 30–50% during pregnancy, with evidence of reduced levels in the first trimester in some individuals. This occurs despite a diet adequate in vitamin B_{12} and is likely to be due to a combination of increasing maternal plasma volume, hormonal changes, increasing maternal requirement and vitamin B_{12} transfer to the fetus. Overall, the bulk of current evidence suggests that serum or plasma homocysteine falls with increasing gestation in most subjects. The impact of folate repletion on these changes, however, requires further investigation.

Although vitamin B_6 indices seem to decrease during pregnancy, it is not clear whether normal pregnancy is associated with a vitamin-B_6-deficient state or not, and, even if it is, whether this has any clinical significance or not. In non-supplemented pregnancies there is a progressive fall in serum folate with increasing gestation and either a rise, or no change, in red cell folate can both occur.

Hemostasis

Pregnancy is associated with significant changes in hemostasis. An understanding of the normal hemostatic system and these physiological changes is essential to the diagnosis and management of bleeding and thrombotic disorders. It is also necessary to understand the limitations of the D-dimer algorithms that are used in the screening of non-pregnant subjects suspected of venous thromboembolism (VTE). Furthermore, it may provide an insight into the mechanisms of not only gestational venous thrombosis, but also pregnancy loss and complications such as pre-eclampsia, which have recently been associated with both acquired and heritable thrombophilia.

Pregnancy results in an upregulation in the maternal coagulation cascade, which leads to an overall increase in thrombin generation. This maternal alteration in coagulation is clearly a physiological preparation for delivery. As with many biological factors, this change in coagulation factors may relate to alterations in: hormone-influenced synthesis; the volume of distribution; lipid interaction; or catabolism. The progressive increase in maternal estrogen levels may alter the uptake of coagulation proteins into the uterus and may also result in an increase in the uterine generation of tissue factor. It is possible that both placental and maternal thrombin have an important influence on cellular growth, and thrombin generation results in fibrin formation, which is essential for placental implantation.

Normal hemostasis control

Coagulation

Upon damage to the endothelium, platelets adhere to the subendothelium and activation of the coagulation cascade occurs (Figure 1.1). This results in the combination of a platelet plug and fibrin mesh formation at the site of injury. There are, of course, substantial controls to limit thrombosis to sites of injury and prevent excessive clot formation. Two cascades are still described in blood coagulation. These are the intrinsic and the extrinsic pathways. It is now apparent that the intrinsic pathway (which is activated when blood comes into contact with a negatively charged surface) acts to amplify the coagulation activation occurring as a consequence of the extrinsic pathway.

In the extrinsic pathway, when vascular injury occurs, cells (including endothelial cells and monocytes) express tissue factor (TF), a membrane-bound protein (which is also known as thromboplastin). When this is exposed to plasma, a complex of TF and the plasma serine protease, Factor (F) VII is formed. TF acts as a cofactor for activated FVII and is the most potent known initiator of the coagulation pathway. Ninety-nine per cent of FVII circulates in the zymogen or unactivated form (FVIIc)

Figure 1.1 The coagulation cascade

The 'extrinsic' initiation of coagulation with a combination of tissue factor (TF), Factor (F) VII and activated FVII (FVIIa) is shown. Solid lines indicate activation and dotted lines indicate inhibition; the principal pathway is shown in bold type. The FVII–FVIIa–TF complex activates FX (X) to FXa (Xa), as well as FIX (IX) to FIXa (XIa): this results in the activation of prothrombin (PT) in a prothrombinase complex of calcium (Ca^{2+}), phospholipid (Plipid) and activated FV (Va), resulting in a burst of thrombin. This burst of thrombin activates FV (V) to FVa (Va), FVIII (VIII) to FVIIIa (VIIIa) and FXI (XI) to FXIa (XIa). The combination of thrombin's action and activation of the 'intrinsic' coagulation pathway by exposure to damaged endothelium (via activation of FXII (XII) to FXIIa (XIIa), results in activation of FXI (XI); this leads to activation of FIX (IX). The further activation of FX (X) in the Tenase complex of FIXa (IXa), FVIIIa (VIIIa), Plipid and Ca^{2+} amplifies the coagulation initiated by the thrombin burst. Thrombin also activates FXIII (XIII), which cross-links and stabilizes formed fibrin.

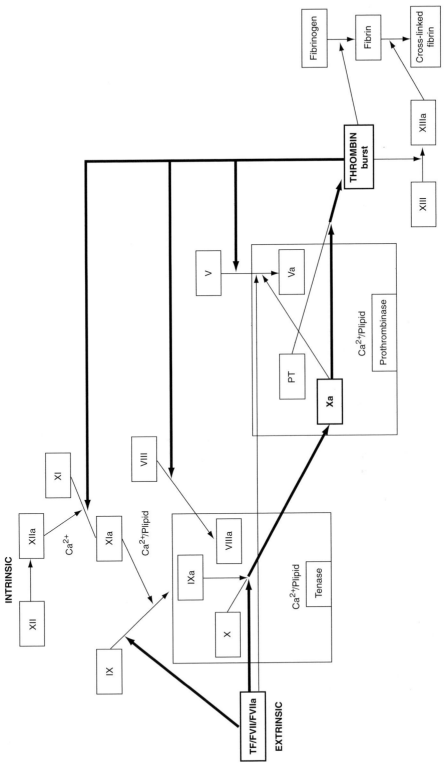

and around 1% circulates as FVIIa, the activated form. Both FVIIc and FVIIa are bound to TF expressed on the vessel wall and inflammatory cells, thereby localizing the hemostatic response to the site of injury. Once FVIIc binds to TF it can be activated by TF itself. This complex can convert further FIXc to FIXa, FXc to FXa, and FVc to FVa. Formed FXa binds to FVa to form a complex (the prothrombinase complex) with calcium on a phospholipid membrane surface. In the presence of these phospholipids, further FVc is converted to FVa and prothrombin is activated leading to a 'thrombin burst'. As prothrombin is cleaved by FXa to form thrombin, a fragment is released. This fragment is called prothrombin fragment 1+2 (F1+2) and, measured in plasma, can be used as a measure of thrombin generation. The thrombin burst can then convert fibrinogen to fibrin, and activate parts of the intrinsic pathway (FVIIIc and FXIc), as well as FVc, FXIIIc (which leads to cross-linking and stabilization of formed fibrin), the endothelium, platelets and monocytes. As thrombin is also involved in anticoagulation and fibrinolysis (see below), it has a central role in orchestrating the hemostatic response.

In the intrinsic pathway, the binding of FXIIc to a negatively charged surface leads to a local increase in FXIIc concentration, which results in its autoactivation. FXIIa causes the conversion of pre-kallikrein to kallikrein, and activates FXIc to FXIa. FXIa, as well as the TF–FVIIa complex, activates FIX to FIXa. Activated FIXa forms a complex (the Tenase complex) with FVIIIa, calcium and phospholipids. This results in activation of FXc to FXa, which contributes to the prothrombinase complex and further thrombin generation.

Thrombin converts soluble fibrinogen to an insoluble fibrin polymer, which seals the site of injury and protects damaged tissue during wound healing. Fibrinogen activation generates soluble fibrin monomers, fibrinopeptide A and fibrinopeptide B. The resultant fibrin mesh is stabilized by cross-linking catalyzed by thrombin-activated coagulation FXIIIa.

Coagulation control

There are a number of controls of coagulation (Figure 1.2). TF pathway inhibitor (TFPI) is released constitutively from endothelial cells, and, in associ-

Figure 1.2 Coagulation control

The principal points of physiological inhibition and downregulation of the coagulation cascade are shown. Solid lines indicate a positive effect and dotted lines indicate inhibition. The main inhibitors are antithrombin (AT – previously called antithrombin III). AT inhibits almost all of the coagulation factors, but its principal targets are Factor (F) Xa and thrombin. The interaction of AT with thrombin results in the formation of the thrombin–antithrombin (TAT) complex. Thrombin, when it binds to endothelial thrombomodulin (TM), loses its procoagulant activity and activates protein C (PC) to activated protein C (aPC). aPC, with its cofactor protein S (PS), cleaves activated FV (Va) and activated FVIII (VIIIa). PC can also be activated independently by the endothelial protein C receptor (EPCR). Other inhibitors of coagulation include tissue factor pathway inhibitor (TFPI), which rapidly inactivates the FVII–FVIIa–tissue factor (TF) complex. In addition, antitrypsin and C_1-esterase inhibitor are capable of inhibiting FXIa and FXIIa respectively. Ca^{2+}, Calcium; Plipid, phospholipid.

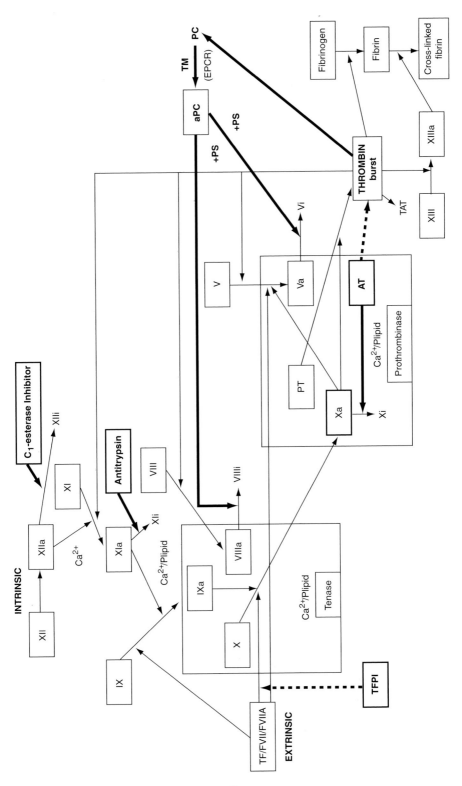

ation with FXa, is able to rapidly inactivate the TF–FVIIa complex. Other controls include antithrombin, which can inhibit many activated clotting factors including thrombin and FXa. By binding to antithrombin, thrombin forms a stable thrombin–antithrombin (TAT) complex, which is rapidly cleared from the circulation. Another regulatory mechanism is protein C, which circulates as an inactive zymogen. To become activated it binds to the endothelial protein C receptor (EPCR), or the transmembrane protein thrombomodulin, which is expressed on endothelial cells. The formation of a thrombin–thrombomodulin complex on the endothelial surface accelerates thrombin's activation of the natural anticoagulant protein C by around 20 000-fold. Formation of this complex directly inhibits the capacity of thrombin to cleave fibrinogen and activate platelets. To function as an inhibitor, activated protein C (aPC) dissociates from EPCR and binds to its cofactor protein S. Protein S has no enzymatic activity of its own, but acts as a cofactor to aPC in the inactivation of FVa and FVIIIa. This then results in a marked reduction in activity of the prothrombinase complex.

Additional inhibitors include the complement component C1-esterase inhibitor (which inhibits FXIIa) and antitrypsin (which can inhibit factor FXIa). In addition, α_2-macroglobulin acts as a broad-spectrum proteinase inhibitor, which has a secondary function to other proteinases and may also be involved in the regulation of the immune system.

Fibrinolysis

Additional clotting control comes from lysis of the fibrin clot (Figure 1.3). Fibrinolysis results from a series of enzymes that control the cleavage of fibrin. These include plasminogen, which when activated by plasminogen activators results in plasmin. This lyses fibrin to fibrin degradation products (including D-dimers). The major activator of plasminogen is tissue plasminogen activator (tPA) – a serine protease produced by endothelial cells – but FXIIa, FXIa, kallikrein and

Figure 1.3 Fibrinolysis

The action and principal controls of fibrin breakdown (fibrinolysis) are shown. Solid lines indicate activation and dotted lines indicate inhibition. Tissue plasminogen activator (t-PA) activates plasminogen to plasmin, which can break down both fibrin and fibrinogen. This results in the generation of a number of fibrinogen and fibrin degradation products, which can have an overall inhibitory effect on further fibrin clot generation. Products released from fibrinogen include D and E fragments, and products released from formed, cross-linked fibrin include D-dimer, Y-dimer and DY fragments. t-PA is, in turn, inhibited and controlled by plasminogen activator inhibitor (PAI)-1. In pregnancy the placenta produces PAI-2, although it does not have a major function in the control of fibrinolysis in the mother. Plasmin is principally inhibited by α-2 antiplasmin, although there is a contribution from α-2 macroglobulin. Thrombin is also capable of the activation of thrombin activatable fibrinolysis inhibitor (TAFI), which inhibits the action of plasmin on formed fibrin. In addition, urokinase (u-PA), which is found in urine, can activate plasminogen. uPA itself is activated from pre-u-PA after limited hydrolysis by kallikrien, which is derived from the intrinsic pathway of coagulation.

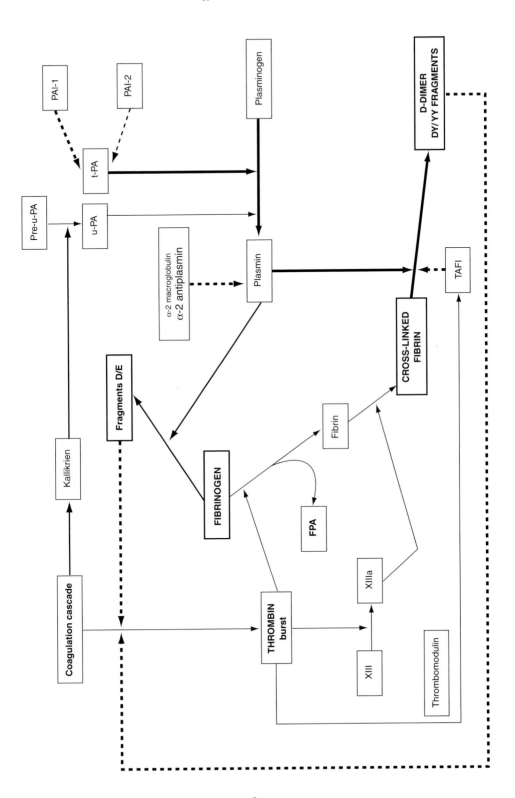

urokinase (uPA) are also capable of activating plasminogen. Release of tPA from the endothelium near the site of injury may result from the action of fibrin, by thrombin attached to the fibrin clot or by the effect of venous occlusion itself. The primary inhibitor of plasmin is α_2-antiplasmin. Other potential plasmin inhibitors include α_2-macroglobulin, antithrombin, α_1-antitrypsin and C_1-esterase inhibitor. In addition, there are four plasminogen activator inhibitors of which plasminogen activator inhibitor (PAI)-1 is the most important in vivo. PAI-1 is released from the endothelium in response to agents such as thrombin and endotoxin. PAI-2 is produced only in the placenta and so is only found in pregnant women. In addition to these controls, thrombin, when bound to thrombomodulin, can activate thrombin-activatable fibrinolysis inhibitor (TAFI). TAFI cleaves the COOH terminal end of fibrin. This reduces the ability of fibrin to facilitate plasminogen activation via tPA. TAFI also directly inhibits plasmin activity and, when cross-linked to fibrin, prevents premature lysis.

Pregnancy-associated changes in coagulation and fibrinolysis

Coagulation

Increasing gestation is associated with a progressive increase in the plasma concentrations of fibrinogen, FVIIc, FVIIIc, FXc and FXIIc, von Willebrand factor (vWF) antigen and the functional measure of vWF, ristocetin cofactor activity (see Chapter 4). No consistent change in FVc and FIXc is seen, but a reduction in FXIc is likely (Table 1.2). Despite the large number of longitudinal and cross-sectional studies of hemostasis in normal pregnancy, the mechanism and significance of these changes remain poorly understood. An increase in TAT complex formation occurs in normal pregnancy, and TAT complex levels higher than non-pregnant control values have been reported to be present in 50% of women during the first trimester, with all subjects showing elevated levels in the second and third trimesters. A significant positive correlation between gestational stage and F1+2 has also been shown, with levels elevated beyond non-pregnant subjects seen early in pregnancy. In addition, pregnant plasma, in in vitro experiments, is capable of more rapid and elevated generation of thrombin than non-pregnant plasma. This, in combination with evidence of an increase in prothrombin activation and TAT complex formation (in the absence of any increase in antithrombin levels) suggests that a heightened thrombin generation potential may be a feature of normal pregnancy and, it has been suggested, may indicate a prothrombotic state.

Coagulation control in pregnancy

A number of studies have shown no difference in protein C antigen, or activity, when pregnant subjects were compared with those who were not pregnant. In most studies, no effect of increasing gestation on protein C (activity or antigen levels) or antithrombin levels has been observed (Table 1.3).

Table 1.2 – Coagulation in pregnancy

	Change from first to second trimester (%)	Change from first to third trimester (%)
Fibrinogen	↑ 11	↑ 31
Prothrombin	0	0
FVc	0	0
FVIIc	↑ 16	↑ 42
FVIIIc	↑ 28	↑ 62
FIXc	0	0
FXc	↑ 15	↑ 20
FXIc	↓ 5	↓ 5
FXIIc	↑ 16	↑ 14
vWF antigen	↑ 22	↑ 96
TAT	↑ 82	↑ 128
F1+2	↑ 80	↑ 140
FPA	↑ 83	↑ 80
D-dimer	↑ 170	↑ 180
Soluble fibrin	↑ 26	↑ 45

F, Factor; FPA, Fibrinopeptide A; TAT, Thrombin–antithrombin complex; vWF, von Willebrand Factor.

Pregnancy results in a fall in free and total protein S levels, with levels less than those of non-pregnant subjects observed in the first trimester, and levels <50% of those observed in the first trimester evident between 36 and 40 weeks gestation.

Table 1.3 – Coagulation control in pregnancy

	Change from first to second trimester (%)	Change from first to third trimester (%)
Protein C activity	0	0
Protein C antigen	0	0
Antithrombin activity	0	0
Protein S total	↓ 9	↓ 15
Protein S free	↓ 20	↓ 30
Plasma thrombomodulin	↑ 10	↑ 41
APTT–APCR	↑ 13	↑ 20
Modified APTT–APCR	0	0

aPCR, Activated protein C resistance; APTT, Activated partial thromboplastin time.

As is discussed in Chapter 7, the significance of inherited resistance to aPC (aPCR) was recognized by Dahlback and co-workers in 1993 (Dahlback B, et al 1993). In the majority of subjects, inherited resistance is due to the Leiden mutation in the gene coding for coagulation FV (FV Leiden). Pregnancy is associated with a progressive increase in aPCR, which is independent of the Leiden mutation. This resistance can be assessed by activated partial thromboplastin time (APTT) or TF-based assays (see below). In APTT-based methods, the results are reported as a sensitivity ratio (which is inversely related to the degree of resistance). Modification of these assays by pre-dilution of the patient plasma with FV-deficient plasma renders the tests highly specific for the mutations in the FV gene, and insensitive to acquired aPC resistance or the effects of pregnancy.

Thrombomodulin, as noted above, is found on maternal vascular endothelial cells and on the trophoblastic surface of the placenta. A soluble form of thrombomodulin exists in plasma and urine, and has been widely used as a marker of endothelial damage. Normal pregnancy may be associated with an increase in soluble thrombomodulin levels, but the relationship between this cleaved form and the overall anticoagulant effect of thrombin (via aPC generation) is unknown. aPC is known to be regulated by several inhibitors, including protein C inhibitor-1, α_1-antitrypsin, α_2-antiplasmin, C_1 esterase inhibitor and α_2-macroglobulin. It is possible to assess the activity of thrombin on protein C activation by measuring aPC, by measuring the peptide released from protein C on activation, or by measuring complexes of aPC with its inhibitor α_1-antitrypsin. An increase in aPC–α_1-antitrypsin in the third trimester to near double the level of that observed in the first trimester occurs in normal pregnancy. This does not correlate with α_1-antitrypsin, suggesting that increasing gestation is associated with an increase in the activation of protein C and therefore an increase in thrombin-mediated antithrombotic activity.

The overall balance of the prothrombotic and antithrombotic effects of thrombin has not been clarified, but higher levels of fibrinopeptide A (a fragment released on the activation of fibrinogen), are also a feature of pregnancy, indicating that there is a parallel increase in fibrin generation.

Fibrinolysis

The activation and inhibition of fibrinolysis occurs at a local level, so the study of plasma can only give a limited insight into the balance of fibrinolysis during pregnancy. Increasing gestation is associated with a complex alteration in plasma markers of plasminogen activation and inhibition. Plasminogen activity, and PAI-1 and PAI-2 levels increase throughout pregnancy. This is accompanied by a probable increase in tPA antigen but a reduction in its activity and release after venous occlusion. No alteration in α_2-antiplasmin levels has been reported in normal pregnant subjects. A number of studies have shown that increasing gestation is associated with an overall reduction in systemic fibrinolytic activity. Despite this, pregnancy is associated with an increase in circulating fibrin degradation products. The reason for this apparent disparity is not known, although it may point to an increase in fibrin generation and degradation in the placenta (despite a reduction in the fibrinolytic potential of the general circulation), or to a reduction in the plasma clearance of these products.

Delivery and the early puerperium

There are very few studies that have systematically examined the longitudinal changes in coagulation that occur during labor and delivery. Many coagulation factors show little change during labor, but a fall in fibrinogen levels, with a nadir evident at the delivery of the placenta occurs. Levels then rise, perhaps as early as 3 hours after delivery, toward antenatal values. Fibrin degradation products are elevated in early labor, fall during placental delivery and rise immediately again (along with soluble fibrin and D-dimer and fibrinopeptide A levels), indicating an alteration in intravascular coagulation. Whether there is a detectable alteration in the overall ex vivo fibrinolytic activity of maternal plasma evident in the first few hours after delivery is unclear.

No change in total protein S levels during delivery has been reported and a gradual return to non-pregnant levels of both free and total protein S becomes evident in the first week of the puerperium. The effect of delivery on protein C is not fully understood. Maternal plasma antigen levels may fall during the delivery prior to the clamping of the placental cord, rising again after clamping. The duration of any elevation in levels is unclear, as elevated levels of protein C antigen and activity may occur in the first 3–5 days after delivery, but levels may also fall, or remain unchanged. Further study is required to clarify the influence of delivery on protein C levels. Higher acquired aPC resistance, when compared with non-pregnant subjects, does occur at delivery and a return towards non-pregnant values is seen in the first week after delivery.

In the first postpartum week, no reduction (and perhaps a further elevation) of fibrinogen levels from third trimester values is seen in longitudinal investigations. This may be accompanied by a slight rise from antenatal levels in FVc and FXIc. A fall from antenatal levels of FVIIIc and FVIIc is evident between 1 and 7 postpartum days. In the first week of the puerperium, thrombin generation, soluble fibrin levels and D-dimer formation remain higher than in early pregnancy. The first postpartum week is also associated with a fall, from antenatal values, in plasma plasminogen and (consistent with a substantial placental origin) in PAI levels.

Changes in other coagulation assays during pregnancy

The partial thromboplastin time (PTT) measures the intrinsic pathway of coagulation and is so called because the coagulation activator used is phospholipid. By contrast, the prothrombin time (PT) is activated by 'complete' thromboplastin: a mixture of TF and phospholipid. There is considerable variation in the lipid composition of the phospholipid used in different partial thromboplastin tests. This means that each test will vary slightly in its interaction with the clotting factors in the sample being tested. In addition, an activator is used to improve consistency of the assay. Such activators include substances such as kaolin, silica, celite and ellagic acid. To perform this APTT, the patient blood sample is taken into citrate anticoagulant (which chelates ionized calcium, preventing coagulation). The partial thromboplastin and activator are added along with calcium and the time taken for fibrin clot to form is recorded.

PT is a measure of the extrinsic coagulation pathway and is the time taken for a citrated sample of blood to form visible fibrin clot after the addition of calcium and animal-derived TF to the sample.

In most studies of pregnancy, no marked change in the PT occurs with increasing gestation. However, the APTT may shorten (depending upon the test) by up to 4 seconds towards the end of pregnancy, and is also shortened following a recent VTE or surgery. In pregnancy this shortening is likely to be due to the marked physiological increase in FVIIIc, which occurs with increasing gestation. This foreshortening should also be considered when monitoring unfractionated heparin.

Similarly, although low-molecular-weight heparin (LMWH) dosing is often based on non-pregnant kinetics, recent work suggests that pregnancy may result in a later peak of anti-Xa levels (using prophylactic doses) than that found in non-pregnant subjects (4 hours as opposed to 2 hours). Increasing gestation appears to be associated with a reduction in anti-Xa levels.

References

Dahlback B, Carlsson M, Svensson PJ, Proc Natl Acad Sci USA 1993; 90(3):1004–8.

CHAPTER 2

Blood group serology and blood products

Blood transfusion

There are 23 blood group systems that are coded by single or closely linked genes. The genes for the *ABO* and Lewis systems code for enzymes (glycosyltransferases), which transfer sugar molecules onto a carbohydrate chain on the red cell and other tissues. On the red cell, these *A* and *B* enzymes add sugars to the group *O* substance (more properly called the *H* antigen) to form blood groups *A* and *B*, respectively, or, in combination, group *AB*. The expression of these antigens on the surface of red cells and platelets is important, as they can lead to the formation of destructive alloantibodies when presented to antigen-negative subjects. The presence of *ABO* substances on endothelial and epithelial membranes can also lead to problems with solid organ and stem cell transplants.

Forty-two per cent of Caucasians and 36% of Black subjects are group *A*, with 16 and 25% of Caucasians group *B* or *AB*, respectively; the remainder are group *O*. In addition, there are a number of *A*, *B* and *O* antigen subtypes. For example, individuals typed by standard serology as group *A* can be further genetically subtyped as A_1A_1, A_1A_2, A_1O, A_2A_2 or A_2O. Indeed, the majority of group *A* subjects are in fact A_1O. Rarely, some individuals cannot form the *O* (*H*) precursor (the so-called Bombay phenotype), and as a result develop naturally occurring anti-*A*, -*B* and -*H* (*O*) antibodies, making transfusion almost impossible.

In 80% of Caucasians the secretor gene (*Se*) on chromosome 19 also codes for a glycosyltransferase. This leads to secretion of free *A* or *B* substances into plasma and secretions.

The clinical significance of any particular red cell antigen depends upon: the frequency of the antigen; the ease of antibody development to it; the amount of antigen exposure in an antigen-negative subject; and the destructive capacity of the antibody (which depends upon its type, its thermal range and its ability to bind complement or cross the placenta). In general, antibodies of the immunoglobulin (IgM) M class bind complement more readily than IgG. IgM antibodies to groups *A* or *B* occur naturally in subjects who do not carry *A* or *B*, and are thought to arise from natural exposure to an unknown substance that is antigenically similar to the *A* or *B* antigens. IgM antibodies, unlike IgG, do not cross the placenta.

Antibodies formed after exposure to a previously 'unseen' antigen (usually as a consequence of transfusion or pregnancy) are usually of the IgG class. When there has been a previous exposure, re-exposure may result in an anamnestic response (a rapid rise in antibody titer), which is the mechanism behind a delayed transfusion reaction.

Some individuals, such as those with autoimmune disorders or sickle-cell disease, appear more susceptible to the production of red cell antibodies. In contrast, individuals with acquired, physiological (i.e. neonates), or congenital hypogammaglobulinemia, appear to have a reduced susceptibility.

Blood component therapy

To ensure the effective use of donated blood and to provide plasma for fractionation, blood is prescribed as its components: red cells; platelets; fresh frozen plasma (FFP); cryoprecipitate; fractionated clotting factor concentrates and immunoglobulins (Table 2.1). In addition, there are a number of human, or recombinant, clotting factors available for the management of hemophilia, thrombophilia and sepsis. These include recombinant Factor (F) VIIa, recombinant antithrombin, human-derived protein C and recombinant activated protein C.

Red cells

Although many transfusion triggers have been proposed, as a general rule, red cells should be used to treat significant hypoxia due to anemia, i.e. anemia causing cardiac or respiratory distress. In certain circumstances, red cell transfusions may also be used for other purposes, such as the suppression of dyserythropoiesis in thalassemia, or the dilution of sickle cells in sickling disorders.

Table 2.1 – Blood component usage

Component	Indications
Red cells	Hypoxia secondary to anemia
Platelets	Thrombocytopenia + bleeding
Fresh frozen plasma (FFP)	PT/APTT prolonged + bleeding
Cryoprecipitate	Hypofibrinogenemia + bleeding Uremia + bleeding
Fibrinogen concentrate	Hypofibrinogenemia + bleeding Placental maintenance
Recombinant Factor VIIa (rFVIIa)	Life-threatening bleeding + no response to conventional coagulation/platelet/surgical therapy

APTT, Activated partial thromboplastin time; PT, Prothrombin time.

Commonly, the transfusion laboratory will perform a 'group-and-save' procedure for uncomplicated deliveries or Cesarean sections. In this, the blood is typed to determine the ABO and Rh groups, and the patient's serum (or plasma) is tested against a panel of red cells to determine the presence of significant allo- or autoantibodies. If antibodies are detected, the laboratory should proceed to identify the antibody and immediately cross-match the patient's plasma so that compatible blood is available. When no antibody is detected, a rapid cross-match (taking around 10–15 minutes) is performed only when blood is required. Although the majority of patients will have no significant antibodies, the presence of an antibody may delay the provision of compatible blood for several hours, and in some cases for several days. In an extreme emergency, ABO and Rh group-specific, or donor blood phenotyped to be compatible with the major hemolytic antigens in the patient, may have to be used.

FFP

FFP contains all the labile clotting factors and is used to correct a coagulation deficiency – identified by prolongation of the prothrombin or partial thromboplastin times – when bleeding is ongoing, or is predictable, e.g. immediately prior to surgery or closed procedures such as liver biopsy, lumbar puncture and epidural anesthesia. As it is a human blood product (with the attendant risks of immunological or infectious complications), it should not be used for fluid replacement and, where possible, single clotting factor deficiencies should be treated with specific virally inactivated fractionated products. It should be remembered that provision of FFP to the patient will require at least 30 minutes to permit thawing of the product and transport from the transfusion laboratory.

The exceptions to the indications noted above are the provision of the protease required in the treatment of thrombotic thrombocytopenic purpura (TTP)/hemolytic uremic syndrome (HUS) (see Chapter 8), and the provision of anticoagulant proteins such as protein S when a specific product is not available. FFP has no role in the reversal of heparin, but can be used in the reversal of warfarin. However, severe bleeding secondary to warfarin will require a prothrombin concentrate, as FFP will not lead to an adequate restoration of plasma FIXc levels in these circumstances.

Cryoprecipitate and Fibrinogen

Cryoprecipitate is used when the plasma fibrinogen is reduced and there is bleeding, or bleeding is likely. In the non-pregnant state, transfusion should be considered when the plasma fibrinogen is <1g/l. In pregnancy there is a physiological rise in plasma fibrinogen with increasing gestation. The threshold for its use in pregnancy may therefore require adjustment to account for these changes (see Chapter 1). In subjects with congenital hypofibrinogenemia, fibrinogen has also been used to maintain the placental integrity. Where a licensed virally inactivated fibrinogen concentrate is available, this should be used when such fibrinogen treatment is required.

Platelets

Platelets are produced either by plasma exchange (where one adult dose is obtained from one donor) or from the buffy coat of whole blood donations (where four donations are required to provide an equivalent adult dose). Platelets are stored at room temperature (specifically $22+/-2°C$) and have a shelf life of 5 days if continually agitated. Platelet transfusions are indicated in the prevention and treatment of bleeding due to thrombocytopenia (a reduced platelet count) or thrombasthenia (a qualitative platelet defect). As with all plasma products, platelets carry the risks of transfusion outlined below. In addition, there is the potential risk of maternal RhD alloimmunization.

Thrombocytopenia can occur for a number of reasons (see Chapter 8). Although, in general, platelets should only be used where bleeding is attended by thrombocytopenia, there is also a role, albeit more limited, for prophylactic use. A threshold for prophylaxis is not evidence based, but there is consensus that a threshold of $10\times10^9/l$ is now acceptable if there are no additional risk factors such as infection, vomiting or coagulopathy. This contrasts with the previous accepted threshold of $20\times10^9/l$. An individual decision on dosing will be required if there is a concern over platelet refractoriness, or if there is immune thrombocytopenia (ITP: when donor platelets may be destroyed in the same way as endogenous platelets), or when the patient has a stable chronic thrombocytopenia.

In non-pregnant subjects, a platelet count of $50\times10^9/l$ has been adopted as the safe minimum for surgical procedures, or when there is major bleeding. With Cesarean sections, a level of at least $80\times10^9/l$ has been recommended to allow epidural anesthesia; for a vaginal delivery (without epidural anesthesia), a level of $50\times10^9/l$ is acceptable. Clearly, in the peripartum patient with thrombocytopenia, non-steroidal analgesics should be avoided. In each instance a check should be made that the appropriate platelet count has been achieved before the commencement of surgery.

In platelet function disorders, medication that interferes with platelet function should be avoided or withdrawn (such as non-steroidal analgesics and aspirin), and the hematocrit should be optimized prior to platelet transfusion. Desmopressin (trade name DDAVP: see Chapter 4) should be considered if there is an inherited platelet defect. As DDAVP is very similar to oxytocin, there was concern that DDAVP might induce uterine contractility. However, it is now known that these agents operate through different receptors and that DDAVP does not cause uterine contractions.

When RhD-positive platelets are transfused to an RhD-negative woman (who is pregnant or in the reproductive age group), a dose of 250 IU of anti-D should be given to cover between 3 and 5 adult doses of RhD-positive platelets in any 6-week period. Where there is thrombocytopenia it can be given subcutaneously. Platelets intended for intrauterine transfusion should be, where possible: <24 hours old; leukodepleted; apheresis derived; cytomegalovirus (CMV) sero-negative and gamma irradiated. These factors will reduce the infusion volume and the risks of infection and transfusion-associated graft versus host disease.

In non-pregnant subjects, dosing formulas can be used to attempt to predict the dose required to achieve a particular platelet increment. In practice, however, it is usual to give a single adult dose (as noted above, derived from one apheresis or four whole blood donors) over a 30 minute period. As noted above, if there is doubt as to efficacy, the platelet increment can be checked at either 1 or 24 hours after dosing.

Immunoglobulin

Intravenous human normal Ig (IVIgG) is used in the management of a number of conditions which can occur in pregnancy. These include ITP, neonatal alloimmune thrombocytopenia (NAIT), post-transfusional purpura (PTP: see Chapter 8), Guillain-Barré syndrome, myesthenia gravis and some cases of hemolytic disease of the newborn (HDN). Although immunoglobulin has also been used in the management of recurrent fetal loss, recent systematic reviews and clinical trials have shown no evidence for this use. However, further information on patient selection and the timing of infusions may yet indicate a subset of patients who may benefit from it.

As with any blood component there is a risk of pathogen transmission, although modern IVIgG should undergo at least two distinct viral inactivation procedures; and furthermore, there is some evidence that the process of fractionation itself leads to a reduction in prion contamination. The most commonly reported significant side effects with IVIgG are fever, acute renal failure, jaundice, thrombosis and a positive direct antiglobulin test (+/− autoimmune hemolysis). However, these problems may also relate to the underlying condition. Acute tubular necrosis appears more common in products containing sucrose, and occurs more frequently in subjects with pre-existing renal disorders or those on nephrotoxic drugs. In such cases a low sucrose product should be used. In all cases, renal function should be checked prior to infusion and monitored in the days after completion. In addition, the maximum dose and dose rate should never be exceeded. Mild hypersensitivity to IVIgG is not uncommon, but severe reactions are rare and may be associated with severe IgA deficiency. There are a number of reports of venous thrombosis, perhaps related to increased plasma viscosity or enhanced platelet aggregation; and there are also reports of cerebral ischemia of arterial origin (CIAO) in association with IVIgG use. The exact risks are, however, hard to define, as no substantial comparative trials of different IVIgG products have ever been carried out.

Recombinant factor VIIa (rFVIIa)

rFVIIa has been used extensively in the management of acquired inhibitors to FVIII. rFVIIa (complexed with tissue factor) generates thrombin, via activation of FX, on activated platelets. At the dose of rFVIIa given therapeutically this reaction is independent of FVIII and FIX. The requirement for exposed tissue factor and activated platelets should, however, limit rFVIIa action to the site of injury. The full thrombin burst generated by therapeutic-dose rFVIIa appears to be sufficient to cause hemostasis in a wide variety of clinical circumstances, including thrombasthenia and thrombocytopenia, although there is, as yet, little clinical trial evidence for its use. The usual dose is 90–120µg/kg given 2–3 hourly; although a full hemostatic effect may be observed after one dose and a useful therapeutic effect may even be achieved at half this dose. The appropriate method of monitoring rFVIIa is not fully defined, but thrombin generation, thromboelastography, or whole blood clotting may prove useful in the future.

At present, the risk of venous thrombosis, myocardial infarction, CIAO and disseminated intravascular coagulation (DIC) – in particular in those with pre-existing liver disease, cardiac disease, or pregnancy – can only be assessed from case reports. However, rFVIIa has been successfully used in the management of post- and antepartum hemorrhage. Although the role of rFVIIa in acquired bleeding disorders is not defined, if it is used in subjects with a severe life-threatening bleeding diathesis (when coagulation screens and bleeding sources have been, or cannot be, corrected by conventional means) there is likely to be a favorable clinical and cost–benefit ratio.

Transfusion in warm autoimmune hemolytic anemia

The provision of compatible blood for patients with autoimmune hemolytic anemia can be significantly problematic. The indications for transfusion, however, are the same as for those without an autoantibody, as the survival of red cells in such patients should be sufficient to improve oxygenation. As with any transfusion, however, red cell compatibility tests should be carried out to exclude the presence of any alloantibody that could cause significant hemolysis of transfused red cells. This is achieved by testing the patient plasma against a panel of donor cells to determine if antibodies to any of these cells are present in the plasma. Some autoantibodies will react against the majority of donor cells, and such a non-specific reaction may mask an alloantibody and make the provision of a compatible transfusion difficult and extremely time consuming.

The presence of an autoantibody is suspected when there is a positive direct antiglobulin (Coombs') test. This indicates the presence of an antibody coating the patient's cells. Although, as noted above, free autoantibodies in the patient plasma often react to all of the cells in a donor panel, occasionally the plasma will react more strongly to some cells than others. This may indicate that the autoantibody has some specificity to one particular antigen, or that an alloantibody is also present. When, as is more often the case, the patient's serum reacts equally against all donor cells, there are a number of strategies to determine if there is also an underlying alloantibody.

If the patient has not received a transfusion within the previous 3 months, then it can be assumed that there will not be significant levels of any previously transfused donor red cells in the patient. In these circumstances, using a whole blood sample, any autoantibody bound to the patient's red cells is removed with an enzyme ('ZZAP'). These 'stripped' cells are then used to adsorb the free autoantibody from a sample of the patient's plasma at 37°C. This process (autoadsorption) is repeated several times to remove as much of any autoantibody from the patient plasma as possible. The resultant plasma is then used against donor cells to determine if any alloantibody is present. Such an autoadsorption procedure requires a considerable sample of the patient's blood.

If there has been a history of transfusion within the previous 3 months then any donor cells still in the patient may bind to the alloantibody, making detection of an alloantibody unreliable. If autoadsorption cannot be carried out, then an attempt to elute the autoantibody from the patient's serum using allogenic red cells with a variety of antigens can be attempted. A combination of reactions will often assist in detecting a significant hemolytic red cell antibody.

One further strategy is to phenotype the patient and select donor blood that carries the same antigens. Ideally, this phenotyping should include the *RhD, C, E, c, e, Kell, Jk^a, Jk^b, Fy^a,* Fy^b, *S* and *s* antigens. However, the presence of an autoantibody that is adherent to the patient's red cells may make such extended phenotyping impossible, and in such cases autoadsorption will be required.

If the patient's autoantibody is only cold acting, then the compatibility test can be carried out strictly at 37°C. In such circumstances, the autoantibody will have no effect on the compatibility procedure. Such patients should, of course, be given their transfusion through a blood warmer.

In extremely urgent circumstances, the appropriate blood for transfusion may have to be selected upon the basis of the 'least reaction' of donor cells against the patient's plasma. This is an extremely unreliable approach and every effort should be made to formally exclude a significant alloantibody. Further, whether such a selection of 'least incompatible' blood (based upon a slight variability in reactivity in testing of the plasma against a variety of donor cells) improves the survival of donor cells in the patient, when an alloantibody has already been excluded, is unknown.

In urgent circumstances, communication between the laboratory and the clinician is vital, as there may often be time to carry out a limited phenotype to improve the safety of the transfusion when time does not permit an auto-adsorption procedure.

Transfusion reactions

Reactions to transfusions can occur for a number of reasons (Table 2.2). Of these, hemolytic reactions are the most clinically important given their potential frequency and severity. Other reactions, such as transfusion-associated graft versus host disease (TA-GVHD: see below), although significant, occur very rarely.

Table 2.2 – Reactions to transfusions

Hemolysis	Antibody in the recipient (acute or delayed) Alteration of the transfused cells: – Excessive heat/freezing – Bacterial contamination – Mixing with intravenous fluids/drugs – Trauma by infusion devices Antibody in a plasma transfusion
Febrile non-hemolytic	Red cell reactions: from recipient white cell antibodies Platelet reactions: from donor white cell cytokines TRALI: Donor HLA antibodies
Allergy	Urticaria/anaphylaxis
Transfusion-associated graft versus host disease (TA-GVHD)	Cytotoxic donor lymphocytes
Post-transfusion purpura	Recipient-derived anti-HPA Abs
Infection	Bacterial: – Environmental: Staphylococci / Pseudomonas – Syphilis (Treponema) – Lyme disease (Borrelia) – Yersinnia/Salmonella – Q fever (Coxiella) Viral – Hepatitis A, B, C or D – HIV – HTLV – EBV, CMV, HHV – Parvovirus Protozoal – Malaria – Chagas' disease – Toxoplasma – Babesia – Leishmania Prion?

CMV, Cytomegalovirus; EBV, Epstein-Barr virus; HHV, Human herpes virus; HLA, Human leukocyte antigen; HPA, Human platelet antigen; HTLV, Human T-cell leukemia/lymphoma virus; TRALI, Transfusion-related acute lung injury.

Hemolytic reactions

These result from the binding of an antibody to a red cell antigen. This leads to opsonization, with or without complement activation, red cell destruction and the activation of inflammation. In acute reactions this occurs within 24 hours whereas, in delayed reactions, this usually occurs within 5–7 days. Acute hemolysis is often mediated by IgM, which efficiently activates complement leading to intravascular destruction, with release of hemoglobin into the circulation and urine. In the delayed reaction, IgG is often the mediator. As a result there may be no, or incomplete, complement activation. In such cases, red cell breakdown usually occurs in the spleen, leading to a fall in blood hemoglobin levels rather than frank intravascular hemolysis. Cytokines may be released as a consequence of both complement and macrophage/monocyte activation.

Antibodies against ABO are the most common cause of acute hemolytic reactions. This most often results from clerical error leading to the misidentification of the unit of red cells for donation, or misidentification of the recipient. Antibodies against A, B, H (O), K (one of the *Kell* group), *Jk^a* (one of the *Kidd* group) and *Le^a* (one of the *Lewis* antigens) are often associated with intravascular hemolysis. Antibodies against the Rh, Duffy or M, N, or S blood group antigens are most often associated with extravascular hemolysis.

In the acute reaction, even a small volume of red cells may be sufficient to trigger hemolysis. The first signs are often patient apprehension, agitation, fever and diffuse abdominal pain. This may lead to breathlessness, shock, disseminated intravascular coagulation and acute renal failure. Immediately upon suspicion of a reaction, the infusion of blood should be stopped. If possible, the unit of blood should be taken down with the administration set still attached, which allows examination of the unit for evidence of bacteriological contamination. Management should follow the principles shown in Table 2.3.

Delayed hemolytic reactions are usually the result of an anamnestic response occurring upon re-exposure to an antigen. Such re-exposure leads to an increase in the level of antibody in the recipient which can result in red cell destruction. This usually leads to asymptomatic coating of the transfused cells with antibody (a positive direct antiglobulin test), but can result in clinically evident hemolysis with fever, jaundice, a falling hemoglobin level and spherocytosis. This is usually clinically evident some 5–7 days after the transfusion. Although multiple antibodies can be involved, Rh group, Kell, Duffy and Kidd antibodies are most often implicated. Repeat testing some days after the transfusion may be required to detect the antibody. Severe reactions are uncommon and specific treatment, other than the provision of suitable antigen-negative transfusion for continuing anemia, is seldom required.

Non-hemolytic febrile reactions

Non-hemolytic febrile reactions occurring with red cell transfusions are not uncommon. They are caused by pre-formed anti human leukocyte antigen (anti-

Table 2.3 – Management of transfusion reactions

Severe hemolysis?		Stop infusion New venous access Re-examine component for evidence of infection/hemolysis	
	Immediate	Monitor	Temperature Blood pressure Pulse Urine output
		Intravenous fluids	Maintain blood pressure + urine output
		Confirm identity	Wrist band Component label Compatibility form
		Alert transfusion lab	Do not use other cross-matched units until advised by transfusion lab Repeat blood group and antibody screen Lab to repeat pre-screening
	Further tests	Full blood count	Anemia Fragmentation Spherocytes
		Urinalysis	Hemoglobinuria
		Urea and electrolytes	Renal function
		Coagulation screening	Disseminated intravascular coagulation (DIC)
		Blood cultures	Sepsis
		Evidence of Hemolysis	Reticulocytes Haptoglobin Plasma hemoglobin
	Other measures	Dialysis Disseminated intravascular coagulation (DIC) management	(if required)
Fever only		Paracetamol Monitor vital signs	
		Transfusion lab	Advice on restarting
Urticarial			Chlorpheniramine

HLA), or granulocyte-specific, antibodies in the recipient of the transfusion, which react with white cells in the transfused component. Fever and tachycardia can commence within 30 minutes of the beginning of the transfusion, which usually settles within a few hours of cessation. Symptoms may be more severe when transfusion is rapid and the incidence is much reduced by pre-transfusion leukodepletion of the blood component. The principal importance of these reactions is their correct distinction from a more severe hemolytic transfusion reaction, or from bacterial contamination of the blood component. Accordingly, such reactions will often necessitate cessation of the transfusion. Febrile non-hemolytic reactions most often occur during platelet transfusions, in perhaps as many as 40%, when they are likely to be mediated by leakage of inflammatory cytokines from white cells in the platelet component. The universal leukodepletion of blood components in the UK has resulted in a four-fold reduction in the occurrence of such reactions.

Allergy

Mild allergic reactions, such as urticaria and wheeze, are not uncommon with the transfusion of blood components, and may occur after single or multiple exposure. Although often difficult to disentangle from a reaction to concomitant therapies, their immediate management is akin to that of other allergic reactions. Of note, is the rare occurrence of severe IgA deficiency (IgA <0.05mg/dl) in the recipient. This may trigger a reaction on exposure to donor IgA. The detection of specific anti-IgA antibodies in the recipient may assist in making the diagnosis, and such individuals may require washed red cells (which removes the IgA) or consideration for blood-sparing modalities such as cell salvage or autologous donation.

Transfusion-related acute lung injury

Transfusion-related acute lung injury (TRALI) is a relatively rare (around 0.02% of transfusion events), but potentially serious, consequence of transfusion. It is caused by the transfusion of HLA antibodies (within a blood component), which react with the recipient's white cells. The donors are often multiparous women who have formed these antibodies during previous pregnancies and any transfusion component containing plasma can be the source. The antibodies react with the patient's white cells resulting in leukostasis and inflammation within the lung. The patient classically presents a few hours after transfusion with respiratory distress, fever, hypoxia and evidence of bilateral infiltration on the chest X-ray. It may be more common in subjects with sepsis and can be difficult to distinguish from other causes of adult respiratory distress. In 50% of cases, HLA or specific granulocyte antibodies can be detected in the implicated donor plasma. Although mortality may be as high as 1 in 20, with adequate and prompt ventilatory support, resolution occurs in the majority within 7 days of onset. In many countries, strategies to reduce TRALI – plasma reduction of products, screening of female donors for selected antibodies, or exclusion of parous women from plasma-rich component donation – are being considered to reduce the risk. The deferral of blood donors who have received a blood transfusion could also be expected to reduce TRALI risk.

TA-GVHD

TA-GVHD is a very rare, but almost universally fatal, condition caused by the infusion (in a transfusion component) of immune competent lymphocytes. These cells are able to mount an immunological reaction against the recipient. This most commonly occurs in those recipients who share an HLA haplotype with the donor. However, immunodeficiency or immunosuppression in the recipient also predispose to the condition. Patients often present with a rash, diarrhea and abnormal liver function. This progresses to marrow failure and sepsis within 4 weeks of diagnosis. Although there is no specific treatment for the condition, it can be effectively prevented by gamma irradiation of cellular trans-fusion components prior to transfusion.

PTP

Around 2% of Caucasians do not carry the platelet antigen HPA-1a on their platelets and PTP usually occurs in parous women who do not carry this antigen (see Chapter 8). It is assumed in such cases that the mother has carried an HPA-1a positive fetus in a previous pregnancy that has resulted in immunization of the mother, but has not led to the development of neonatal alloimmune thrombocy-topenia (see Chapter 8). Subsequent exposure to the HPA-1a antigen, via a red cell transfusion, results in an increase in the titer of anti-HPA-1a antibodies. This leads, by an essentially unknown mechanism, to destruction of the women's platelets (despite the fact that they do not carry the HPA-1a antigen). This often results in a rapid fall in platelet count presenting around 1 week after the trans-fusion. The resultant thrombocytopenia results in widespread bruising and bleeding from the gastrointestinal or renal tracts.

The condition is diagnosed by the history of recent transfusion and the detec-tion of anti-HPA-1a antibodies in the recipient's serum and exclusion of other causes of thrombocytopenia (see Chapter 8).

Other HPA antibodies have also been reported in association with PTP, including anti-HPA-1b, -3a, -3b, -4a or -5b. As further donor platelets (even if antigen negative) will also be destroyed, platelet therapy may be ineffective. Indeed, there is no evidence that the specific HPA antigen-negative platelets will be more effective than random platelets. So therapy is geared towards suppres-sion of the immune response with high-dose IVIgG therapy. A number of successes have also been reported with plasma exchange. The provision of blood component therapy after an episode can also be problematic, as a recur-rence is unpredictable. It is usual practice to attempt to provide appropriate HPA negative blood for future transfusions, although there may also be a role for leukodepletion or autologous donation.

Bacterial contamination

Bacterial contamination may be present in as many as 1 in 3000 cellular blood component transfusions and, when severe, presents as an acute hemolytic transfusion reaction. The true incidence is difficult to judge, as minor contamination may not lead to clinical problems. Around 60% of fatalities are associated with microbial contamination of platelets.

The primary source of bacterial contamination of blood products is the donor. This can be due to poor cleaning technique at the venesection, or asymptomatic bacteremia in the donor (such as occurs after dental treatment). On account of this, bacterial contamination is also a problem with pre-deposit autologous donation. Problems can be reduced by: taking an adequate donor history; meticulous venesection technique; specific systems to detect microorganisms in blood components; and inspection of the blood component prior to transfusion.

As red cell components are stored at $4°C$, Gram-negative organisms such as Yersinnia and Pseudomonas are often implicated. By contrast, as platelets are stored at room temperature, Gram-positive organisms such as staphlyococci and streptococci are often the cause of such contamination.

New variant Creutzfeldt-Jakob disease (nvCJD)

nvCJD is one of a group of neurodegenerative disorders caused by infection with a prion protein. The mechanism of the disease is not fully understood, but evidence suggests that the infectious agent is an abnormal, protease-resistant form (designated PrP^{Sc}, where 'Sc' stands for 'scrapie') of the normal host prion glycoprotein (designated PrP^c), with a strong likelihood that the disease represents a human form of bovine spongiform encephalopathy. Prion diseases are characterized by deposition of abnormal PrP^{Sc} prion protein aggregates in the brain, leading to spongiform degeneration and neuronal loss. The abnormal protein has the same amino acid sequence as its physiological counterpart, but has a different secondary (folded) structure. It is this altered structure that allows the formation of the protease-resistant aggregates. What is remarkable is that the abnormal protein (PrP^{Sc}) interacts with the native protein (PrP^c), leading it also to adopt this abnormal secondary conformation and further the aggregate deposition.

nvCJD is characterized by a relatively rapid onset of neurological degeneration and dementia. Although the prion's full distribution is not known, there is evidence that cellular interactions are essential in concentrating PrP^c to allow its transformation by PrP^{Sc}. PrP^c is highly expressed on a variety of blood cells, lymphoid cells and cellular microparticles, where it may have a physiological role in the protection from oxidative stress. As a consequence of this potential cellular dependency, blood donations in the UK are routinely leukodepleted prior to transfusion.

The scale of the risk to humans by nvCJD is unknown and whether there are a substantial number of individuals incubating and able to transmit the disorder is also not yet known. Although animals have a different tissue distribution of prion proteins to humans, transmission of prion disease by transfusion has been demonstrated in sheep. Furthermore, in 2004, a person who had donated blood in the UK subsequently developed nvCJD. The recipient of his donation also went on to develop nvCJD some time after the transfusion. Although a link cannot be proven, there is the potential that direct introduction of the abnormal prion by transfusion may bypass the protective effects of enzyme degradation that take place if the prion is ingested in infected meat. It is likely, however, that the absolute risk of prion transmission by transfusion is low. There is also likely to be a reduction in blood product contamination with prions if the products have undergone a fractionation process, such as is used in the manufacture of immunoglobulin or clotting factor concentrates.

However, this theoretical risk of prion transmission by transfusion, allied to the absence of a screening test (although many first generation tests are in development) and evidence that the protein is not susceptible to standard viral inactivation procedures, highlights the need to restrict blood product usage to those indications where there is a clear, positive, benefit:risk ratio.

Cell saving

Cell saving encompasses a number of techniques which attempt to reduce exposure to allogenic blood. These techniques include autologous pre-deposit, intraoperative hemodilution and intra- or postoperative cell salvage. A number of other therapies, such as recombinant erythropoietin and antifibrinolytic agents, are also used to reduce allogenic exposure, and a further strategy is the development of useful blood substitutes.

In view of the potential risks of allogenic transfusion there has been considerable interest in the use of cell-saving techniques in relation to delivery and, in particular, Cesarean section. Although techniques such as pre-deposit of autologous blood and intraoperative cell salvage are well tolerated and considered safe in the majority of instances, their use in pregnancy requires due consideration of their potential effects on maternal and fetal wellbeing. In addition, the widespread adoption of these techniques requires clarification of those in whom such interventions would be clinically or cost-effective.

Autologous pre-deposit

There are many case series examining the feasibility of autologous pre-deposit in relation to obstetrics. Most often pre-deposits (equivalent to 1–2 units of red cells) are taken by standard venesection in the third trimester. Although maternal side effects, such as faintness, are well tolerated, the effects of blood loss on the feto-placental unit are not fully understood. Although it may be that there is no effect on cord blood pressure and flow, it has been suggested that venesection of 400ml of maternal blood in the third trimester is associated with a reduction in fetal middle cerebral artery pulsatility in the first 24 hours after the event. In general, to be suitable, women require a hematocrit sufficient (usually >33%) to permit safe venesection. In addition, there has to be a high probability that collected units will be used. Given this, autologous pre-deposit can be justified in those with multiple or difficult red cell alloantibodies (e.g. thalassemia), those in whom bleeding is likely (e.g. where there is a severe bleeding disorder or placenta previa) and those subjects who cannot receive transfusions (e.g. Jehovah's Witnesses, Bombay phenotypes). In most obstetric patients without placenta previa, the need for peripartum transfusion cannot be predicted with sufficient accuracy to justify antepartum pre-deposit, and in studies of feasibility, only 14–34% of subjects with placenta previa were suitable for pre-deposit. Indeed, as with many cell-saving techniques, the use of pre-deposit leads to an overall increase in the likelihood of transfusion. This increase in the likelihood of use of the autologous pre-deposit means that this modality of therapy actually carries a similar risk of both bacterial contamination and of clerical error to that found in allogenic transfusion.

Intraoperative cell salvage

Although intraoperative salvage has been used extensively in vascular, cardiac and orthopedic surgery, its use in Cesarean section has been limited because of the possibility of re-infusion of blood containing fetal red cells and amniotic fluid components (such fetal cell debris, potassium and tissue factor). It has been supposed that this risk will be minimized by commencement of salvage after removal of the feto-placental unit, by washing and leukodepletion of the salvaged cells, and by attention to the potential for maternal RhD immunization. Although these measures should reduce the risk, and although salvage is likely to reduce the risk of allogenic exposure, there have been no studies of adequate power to determine if salvage increases the thrombotic and infection risk to the mother. Given these potential problems, the lack of predictability of obstetric hemorrhage and the reliability of allogenic transfusion in developed countries, salvage should be considered in cases where allogenic transfusion is unacceptable (or technically problematic), and only when there is a high likelihood of transfusion.

Erythropoietin

Erythropoietin (Epo) is a glycoprotein, which is synthesized in the kidney in response to hypoxia. Recombinant human Epo is derived from Chinese hamster ovary cells, and has been used widely in anemia associated with renal failure, malignancy and chemotherapy. It is given subcutaneously, at a dose of 50–200IU/kg two–three times per week along with oral or parenteral iron, with the aim of increasing the hemoglobin by 1g/dl/month. It has been used in Jehovah's Witnesses and in the management of renal failure in pregnant subjects, and appears to be well tolerated. Although it does not cross the placenta, it carries a risk of hypertension, and excessive elevation of hemoglobin may also be associated with thrombosis. At present, Epo has a place in the management of neonatal anemia of prematurity, but its use in maternal anemia, or as an adjunct to autologous or salvage techniques in pregnancy, requires further clinical- and cost-effectiveness evaluation.

Blood substitutes

There is a demand to produce red cell and platelet substitutes to address a combination of concerns. These include shortages in blood supply, the risks of contamination and immunomodulation, the costs associated with blood collection, the cost of temperature-regulated storage, the need for cross-match procedures, and the need for strict patient identification. There has been a substantial advance in the development of solutions able to achieve volume expansion and, although a number of blood substitutes able to carry oxygen are in development, the majority are not yet in clinical use. Such products are required to take up oxygen in the lungs and give it up in the tissues. They are also required to be non-toxic, to have a useful half-life in the body and a useful shelf life for storage.

There has been much attention on hemoglobin-based solutions. Unfortunately, hemoglobin readily participates in redox reactions leading to oxidative damage. As a consequence, free hemoglobin has a short half-life and is a potent vasoconstrictor. A number of attempts to improve the stability of hemoglobin by cross-linking have been attempted. Of these, bovine polymerized hemoglobin has a licence for use in veterinary practice. The different hemoglobin products in current development, however, have differing oxygen affinities, hemoglobin concentrations and stability. The major side effect of these products is hypertension, which results from vasoconstriction (by an as yet poorly defined mechanism, perhaps related to a local reduction in nitric oxide or alteration in viscosity), which may in fact hamper oxygen supply.

One other group of products are the perfluorocarbon emulsions, which take up oxygen to a greater degree than human plasma, but do not have the flexibility of uptake and supply associated with hemoglobin. Perfluorocarbon emulsions may also modulate the inflammatory response, and their use can be associated with the development of flu-like symptoms.

At present, none of the available red cell substitutes offer the immediate prospect of a useful oxygen supply without the risks and costs associated with current transfusion therapies, and there is no specific evidence of their safety in pregnancy.

Hemolytic disease of the newborn

The Rh blood group antigens on red cells result from the action of two related genes which code for RhD and RhC/RhE. These blood groups are inherited as two haplotypes, consisting of a combination of c or C, D or no D, e or E. Of these the most important Rh type in obstetric practice is RhD, which is around 50 times more immunogenic than other Rh types. Fifteen per cent of Caucasians, 5% of Black subjects and 2% of Asians are RhD negative. When an RhD-negative mother is carrying an RhD-positive child, the transplacental passage of both fetal blood and maternal IgG immunoglobulin may result in the development of an anti-RhD antibody in the mother that is also active in the fetus.

Whether the mother develops an antibody depends upon the amount of fetal blood entering the maternal circulation and the presence of any feto-maternal ABO mismatch, which reduces the development of an anti-RhD antibody (presumably by clearance of fetal cells by pre-formed maternal anti-A or anti-B antibodies). The Rh haplotype carried by the fetus may also be important as the fetal carriage of cDE/cde is more likely to induce antibodies than other RhD-positive haplotypes. If an RhD-negative woman carries an ABO-compatible, RhD-positive child there is a one in six chance of forming anti-RhD in the absence of prophylaxis. If an RhD-negative recipient receives an RhD-positive transfusion there is a 90% chance of forming anti-RhD. The majority of hemolytic disease cases occur in the second pregnancy, but in some instances the fetal cells may result in a brisk maternal response leading to significant fetal hemolysis in the first pregnancy.

The amount of RhD expressed on the red cell is dependent upon which other members of the Rh haplotype are present. There are also many other quantitative and qualitative variations in RhD expression. Where there is a reduction in the expression of all RhD epitopes, this is termed 'weak D'. The definition of weak RhD is, however, dependent upon the sensitivity of the local laboratory reagents used to detect RhD. On the other hand, the absence of some of the RhD epitopes is termed 'variant D', and there are many classes of variant D. As someone with a weak D has all the RhD epitopes present, exposure to RhD-positive blood will not result in such an individual developing anti-RhD, and such individuals should be classed as RhD-positive. The importance of detecting weak RhD in blood donors is a matter of debate, but such weak D cells could be capable of eliciting an antibody response in a recipient. On the other hand, if someone has a variant D, they may be capable of developing anti-RhD on exposure to RhD-positive cells (from a fetus or from transfusion). In particular, one type of variant RhD (called RhD[VI]) may, upon exposure to RhD, lead to the development of both anti-RhD and HDN. On account of this, in obstetric practice, the laboratory reagents used for antenatal typing should not detect the RhD[VI] variant, and such mothers should be classed as RhD negative. As such, they should receive RhD-negative blood products and prophylactic RhD immunoglobulin if potential sensitizing events occur (Table 2.4). Whether a transfusion of D[VI] donor blood carries a significant risk of sensitizing a recipient is not clear. In any case, when a laboratory cannot reliably distinguish RhD variants from a weak RhD phenotype, it is safer for the mother to be considered to be RhD-negative.

Table 2.4 – Potential RhD-sensitizing events

Antepartum hemorrhage (Including threatened abortions)	
Abdominal trauma	
Ectopic pregnancy	
Fetal external version	
Delivery	
Invasive investigations	Amniocentesis
	Chorionic villous sampling
	Fetal blood sampling
	Embryo reduction
	Shunt insertion
Fetal loss	Intrauterine death
	Stillbirth
	Miscarriage with evacuation
	Complete or incomplete miscarriage >12 weeks
	Therapeutic termination

There are three general classes of IgG immunoglobulin, each with differing characteristics. Of these, HDN only occurs with IgG of the subclasses IgG_1 or IgG_3, which are capable of transplacental passage. The transplacental passage of IgG_1 may occur as early as 20 weeks gestation, with the peak of IgG_3 evident at around 28 weeks. Despite this, IgG_3 is associated with greater postnatal jaundice than IgG_1. As IgG_1 rarely binds complement, the mechanism of red cell destruction is not clear, but may involve increased presentation of the IgG Fc component to macrophages. The majority of affected fetal red cells are destroyed in the fetal spleen.

Antenatal diagnosis and monitoring

Blood group screening of all women should take place when booking for antenatal care. To determine whether the RhD group is negative, a technique that is sensitive for the presence of weak RhD phenotypes should be employed: circulating maternal anti-RhD is usually detected by an indirect antiglobulin test. Such testing should be repeated routinely at least once between 28 and 32 weeks gestation. In the UK, an estimation between 34 and 36 weeks gestation is also recommended. Where there is a routine antenatal prophylaxis program in place, the testing at 28–32 weeks should be carried out prior to any routine prophylactic dose of anti-RhD being given.

If there has been an antenatal sensitizing event in an RhD-negative woman whether or not she has circulating anti-RhD should be determined, and an estimation of feto-maternal hemorrhage (FMH) carried out (Table 2.5). The presence of any maternal anti-RhD should be determined again at delivery, and a

Table 2.5 – Feto-maternal hemorrhage (FMH) assessment

At delivery around 1 in 200 mothers have an FMH >4ml
< 20 weeks, FMH assessment not required
Assess FMH if mother RhD negative/fetus unknown
Pre-formed immune anti-RhD present, FMH not needed
If not sure if maternal anti-RhD is passive or immune, give standard dose anti-RhD

Maternal blood pattern	Action
Fetal cell +, free RhD –	Assess FMH and give anti-RhD
	Repeat FMH at 48 hours
Fetal cell +, free RhD +	Repeat FMH at 48 hours
Fetal cell –, free RhD +	Do nothing
Fetal cell –, free RhD –	Give standard anti-RhD
	Repeat anti-RhD test at 48 hours

cord blood sample should be obtained to determine the ABO and RhD type of the baby. At delivery, the presence of anti-RhD on the fetal cells should be examined by direct antiglobulin test, and the mother should have a blood sample analyzed for an estimation of FMH.

There is a correlation between the gestation at which antibody is first detected and the severity of any resultant HDN. Therefore, if antibodies are detected at booking, they are likely to cause more problems than those detected for the first time later in pregnancy. If an antibody associated with HDN is detected this should be quantified. For most antibodies this will be achieved by the titer on an indirect antiglobulin test. It has been recognized for some time that automated quantification of anti-RhD antibody levels provides more reproducible and meaningful values than manual titration, with the level of maternal anti-RhD immunoglobulin used to plan further testing and the need for fetal blood sampling or delivery. Indeed, in the case of RhD, it is recommended that the anti-RhD titer should be reported in international units (IU). In general, the absolute value is not as important as any rise in titer with increasing gestation. However, when the levels remains at <4 IU/ml, HDN is unlikely and few fetuses suffer major anemia. In such cases, serial anti-RhD monitoring and ultrasound determination of a combination of parameters (such as Doppler of umbilical vein or middle cerebral artery flow, liver and spleen size, and the early detection of ascites) may assist in management.

When the levels are 4–15IU/ml, there is a moderate risk of HDN and investigation is intituted in some, but not all, areas of the UK. Early in pregnancy, genotyping techniques can be used to genotype the fetus (when the partner is unknown, or it is an RhD heterozygote). Such polymerase chain reaction (PCR) techniques do require due consideration of the ethnic origins of the partners, and both false-positive and false-negative results can occur.

In addition, it is now possible to determine if the fetus is RhD positive (as well as the *Kell* and *c* status: see below) from free fetal DNA obtained from the maternal circulation. Although this is in its infancy, very high sensitivity has been reported in some studies using fluorescence-based PCR techniques.

After 27 weeks gestation, amniocentesis can be used to determine the level of bilirubin in the amniotic fluid by its absorption at 450 nm. The level obtained is interpreted by a Lilley graph – essentially relating the level to a gestation-specific reference range to assist in determining the necessity for intrauterine transfusion or delivery. This technique reflects the degree of fetal hemolysis but not the fetal hemopoietic response, and significant discrepancies between the fetal hematocrit and the amniotic fluid optical density can occur. Analysis of amniotic fluid anti-D concentrations has also been investigated. Although these correlate well with maternal serum anti-D levels, they have no added value in predicting the severity of fetal hemolysis.

As yet, in such cases, fetal assessment by most non-invasive methods, including fetal movement counting, ultrasound appearance and fetal electocardiogram waveforms, have not proved helpful in determining whether the fetus will become anemic. Abnormal fetal heart rate patterns have been described in severe disease, and although cardiotocography (CTG) will identify the seriously anemic fetus it is not sensitive enough to predict mild to moderate anemia. Computerized fetal heart rate analysis has identified a consistent relationship between baseline variability and fetal hematocrit, and warrants further study.

Weekly velocimetry of the fetal middle cerebral artery has also been used to monitor affected fetuses. In such cases, peak systolic velocities >1.5 multiples of the median for the specific gestation have been shown to be predictive of moderate or severe fetal anemia (with 100% sensitivity and a false-positive rate of around 12%), and ultrasound studies correlate well with the bilirubin level in the amniotic fluid. This technique has begun to replace serial amniocentesis and is now being used to predict when fetal blood sampling is required.

The only direct method of assessing the severity of RhD disease, however, is by measuring the hematocrit of fetal blood samples. When levels exceed 15IU/ml or if indicated by velocimetry, fetal blood sampling at >18 weeks gestation may be required. This is not without complications (from <2% mortality in non-affected fetuses to 5–15% fetal mortality in affected cases), and the procedure can result in a marked increase in the maternal antibody levels. Other reported complications include fetal exsanguination, bradycardia, failure to obtain a sample and cord constriction. Fetal blood sampling can be achieved by ultrasound-guided sampling of the cord vessels, the hepatic vein, or the fetal heart, which will also permit an assessment of the fetal RhD group. Fetal blood sampling should only be carried out, however, if there is the expertise and facilities to carry out an intrauterine transfusion, if required.

In summary, when the maternal anti-RhD level is <0.5IU/ml, four-weekly monitoring of anti-RhD levels is all that is required. If anti-RhD levels are >0.5IU/ml, then two-weekly anti-RhD assessment is required. If levels are between 10 and 20IU/ml, fetal blood sampling will usually be required, but the fetus does not often require an intrauterine transfusion. If the maternal anti-RhD level is >20IU/ml, fetal blood sampling will be required and the fetus will probably require intrauterine transfusion. In general, if the anti-RhD level is >4IU/ml but <10IU/ml, then early delivery may be required (however, usually at >36 weeks). For levels of >10IU/ml, 33–38 week delivery may be necessary.

Fetal presentation of HDN

The fetal presentation may be simply with a mild anemia, or in severe cases with a severe anemia, marked jaundice, edema, cardiac failure, widespread effusions and pulmonary hemorrhage. Neurological deficits and seizures (kernicterus) result from passage of bilirubin across the fetal blood–brain barrier. The anemia results in extramedullary hemopoiesis in the liver and spleen. This is associated with a reduction in the production of plasma proteins, which further contributes to the edema. The end result may be stillbirth, neonatal death, or complete resolution.

At birth, a low umbilical venous hemoglobin is seen, although this does not directly equate with disease severity. There is also likely to be a marked reticulocytosis, unless this has been suppressed by recent intrauterine transfusion. The presence of a high concentration of nucleated red cells may result in a factitious high white cell count on automated blood count analyzers.

Fetal management

If fetal maturity permits, delivery of the fetus is indicated when there is evidence of a high level of bilirubin in the amniotic fluid. When fetal immaturity does not make delivery feasible, fetal transfusion should be carried out. The introduction of intrauterine fetal transfusion has reduced the perinatal mortality rate in severe cases of HDN from 95 to 50%. Intrauterine transfusion is indicated if the fetal hematocrit is <25% between 18 and 26 weeks gestation or <30% after 34 weeks gestation. The blood used should be cross-matched against maternal serum and should have a hematocrit of 75–90%, be sero-negative for cytomegalovirus and gamma irradiated. The aim of the transfusion is to increase the fetal hematocrit to around 45%, and the volume required is calculated from the pre-transfusion hematocrit, the donor hematocrit and the estimated fetal blood volume. In some units, pre-medication is given to the mother for maternal and fetal sedation, whilst others have employed tocolytic agents, antibiotics and corticosteroids. The transfusion may be given directly into the fetal vasculature (umbilical vein, umbilical artery, or inferior vena cava), into the fetal heart, or into the fetal peritoneal cavity. Further transfusions may be required at 1–3-weekly intervals. The complications of intrauterine transfusion include transfusion site trauma and hematoma formation, spasm of the cord, umbilical arterial thrombosis, fetal thrombocytopenia, an increase in maternal antibody levels, fetal leukoencephalopathy and fetal bradycardia.

Other modalities of therapy have been used when there has been a history of previous fetal loss, or where the likely father is homozygous for RhD. These include repeated, maternal plasma exchange from early in pregnancy to remove anti-RhD from the maternal circulation until fetal transfusion therapy can be achieved. In such circumstances, maternal procedures, which could cause allo-immunization, should be avoided. Similarly, regular maternal treatment with high-dose human normal immunoglobulin (2g/kg on a two-weekly basis) has also been used in this circumstance.

After delivery, neonatal treatment consists of phototherapy to oxidize bilirubin and, when required, exchange or top-up transfusion.

Prevention

In the 1960s around 46 deaths/100 000 live births were attributed to the RhD immunization in the UK. The routine use of post-delivery anti-RhD immunoglobulin immunoprophylaxis was introduced in 1969. By 1990, the number of fetal deaths attributed to RhD immunization in the UK had fallen to 1.6/100 000. Despite this, there continue to be cases of HDN. This may be due to maternal sensitization in a previous pregnancy, previous transfusion of red cells or platelets, inadequate treatment of potential sensitizing events, sensitization from unrecognized events, or reactions to red cell antigens other than RhD.

Prevention is based upon the suppression of the maternal immune response to the RhD antigen by the timely administration of a passive antibody, the mechanism of which remains poorly understood. Intramuscular anti-RhD should be administered into the deltoid muscle to all RhD-negative women as soon as is practical, but certainly within 72 hours of delivery. If it is not given before 72 hours, every effort should be made to administer it within 9–10 (or even 28) days, as this may still offer some protection. The dose should be determined by the level of FMH. Given intramuscularly, 125IU of anti-RhD is considered sufficient to protect against exposure to 1ml of RhD-positive red cells. In the UK, 250IU is routinely given for any potential sensitizing event that occurs before 20 weeks gestation and 500IU for any event after 20 weeks gestation (see Table 2.4). If a further sensitizing event occurs >7 days after a prophylactic dose of anti-RhD, it is common practice to give a further dose of anti-RhD. In addition, after 20 weeks gestation an FMH assessment should be carried out to determine if the bleed exceeds 4 ml, when a further appropriate dose of anti-RhD may be required (see Table 2.5). It is routine practice in the UK not to give anti-RhD to a threatened miscarriage where the bleeding has stopped before 12 weeks gestation and there is still a continuing pregnancy.

As noted above, some at-risk women may become sensitized in the last trimester by unrecognized events. In fact, given the success of the prophylaxis for sensitizing events, this has become the most important cause of maternal sensitization in many developed countries. One strategy designed to cope with these 'silent' FMH is the routine administration of anti-RhD immunoglobulin to all RhD-negative women who have no detectable anti-RhD antibodies in their blood. This has been shown to further reduce the risk of antenatal immunization. At present, however, a variety of dosages and dosage schedules for prophylaxis have been employed. Of these, two options, which both seem effective, include a dose of 500IU at 28 and 34 weeks gestation or a single larger dose (1500IU) early in the third trimester. Enthusiasm for this method of HDN prevention, however, may be tempered by problems of anti-RhD availability and, in Europe, the continuing concern about the possibility of transmission of prions by blood products, although, as noted above, the process of fractionation is thought to reduce this risk.

Non-RhD antibodies

In addition to RhD, at least 40 red cell antigens have been associated with HDN. These include Rhc, RhC, RhE, Kell, Duffy, MNS, Lutheran, Kidd and U. After anti-RhD, antibodies against c, Kell (K_1) or E are the most frequently encountered antibodies requiring treatment.

Kell

The gene coding for Kell antigens is found on chromosome 7, although expression is also dependent upon genes on the X chromosome. Of the 22 Kell antigens, antibodies to Kell (K_1), k (cellano), Kp^a (Penny), Kp^b (Rautenberg), Js^a (Sutter) and Js^b (Matthews) have all been implicated in HDN. Antibodies to K_1 are the most commonly encountered antibodies after ABO or RhD, and are usually IgG and occasionally complement binding. The K_1 antigen is found in 9% of Caucasians (who are virtually all heterozygous). Kp^b and Js^b antigens have a very high frequency in Caucasians, and Js^b is almost universal in Black subjects. In addition, a reduction in all Kell antigen expression can occur. This is called the Mcleod phenotype and it arises from inheritance of K_x and leads to a chronic mild hemolytic state.

Between 8 and 18% of pregnancies with detectable maternal anti-K_1 result in a K_1-positive fetus, and hydrops has been reported in around 30% of such cases. In recent years this incidence may have been reduced by the use of intrauterine transfusion. In anti-K_1 HDN, fetal anemia results from a combination of hemolysis in the fetal blood as well as destruction in the marrow. This marrow suppression leads to a lower bilirubin level in the amniotic fluid than would be expected by the degree of anemia. The management of a sensitized women requires a combination of ultrasound and fetal blood sampling. One potential strategy in anti-K_1-positive pregnancies is to genotype the father (when paternity can be assured). If the father is kk, no further action may be appropriate. If the father is K_1k, then anti-K_1 titers <4 can be monitored monthly. If a level of 8 is reached, amniocentesis and fetal K_1 typing may be appropriate, as 50% would be expected to be kk. If the fetus is K_1 positive, serial middle cerebral artery Doppler and cordocentesis (with the potential for intrauterine transfusion) should be considered.

In HDN associated with antibodies to *k* (cellano), there may also be an associated reduction in effective red cell production in the marrow, as well as hemolysis within the peripheral blood.

MNS and U

The MNS system is coded on chromosome 4 by two linked genes: GYP A (*M* and *N*) and GYP B (*S*, *s* and *U* alleles). Anti-*M* is relatively common and can be IgG or IgM. Anti *M* can react at $37°C$ and very occasionally has been associated with HDN. There is insufficient data to give specific guidance, but the presence of IgG should be determined, as IgM anti-*M* will not cross the placenta. High IgG titers should lead to further investigation with amniocentesis, and possibly fetal and paternal genotyping. Anti-*N* occurs rarely and is, most often, of no clinical significance.

Both anti-*S* and anti-*s* are usually IgG and have rarely been implicated in HTR or HDN, with the majority of cases of HDN reported resulting in mild hemolysis only. The *U* antigen is essentially only found in Black subjects, and anti *U* is very rare and usually of immune origin. It can be associated, however, with HDN, and geographically where this is a problem, provision of *U*-negative blood for fetal transfusion can be problematic.

Duffy

The Duffy gene consists of co-dominant alleles including *Fy*^{a} and *Fy*^{b}. The Duffy antigen functions as a receptor for *Plasmodium vivax* and carriage of the *Fy*$^{(a-b-)}$ phenotype has been associated with an increased risk of pre-eclampsia, perhaps due to a reduction in Duffy-mediated clearance of interleukin-8.

Antibodies to *Fy*^{a} are more common than *Fy*^{b}, are predominantly IgG and can bind complement. Anti-*Fy*^{b} is not associated with HDN; but HDN associated with anti-*Fy*^{a} has been reported to carry significant morbidity (with one third of cases requiring intrauterine transfusion) and fetal mortality (18% of cases), with significant fetal disease possible at relatively low maternal antibody titers.

Kidd

The Kidd antigens are coded on chromosome 18 and consist of the co-dominant *Jk*^{a} and *Jk*^{b}. Antibodies to *Jk*^{a} are more common than *Jk*^{b}. They usually bind complement and there is often a high percentage of IgG$_3$. Detection of the antibody in maternal plasma can be problematic and often requires the use of homozygous *Jk*^{a} or *Jk*^{b} for detection (i.e. a cell that has homozygote expression of the antigen is required for binding of the maternal antibody to occur). Detection of antibodies may also be complicated by the rapid fall in titers which often occurs soon after an immunization that has arisen as a consequence of transfusion. Anti-Kidd antibodies have been occasionally associated with HDN, and fetal genotyping may assist in determining appropriate care.

Massive obstetric hemorrhage

There are a variety of definitions of major obstetric hemorrhage. These include a requirement to replace 50% of the circulating blood volume (about 6–7l in later pregnancy) in 3 hours, or blood loss requiring the replacement of the whole blood volume (in practice indicated by transfusion of more than 10 units of red cells). Practically, massive blood loss is likely when 1500 ml has been lost. This is often associated with maternal hypotension and should be regarded as a sign of impending massive loss.

It is to be expected that a normal vaginal delivery may involve blood loss of <500 ml and Cesarean section blood loss of up to 1 litre. Although the prediction of massive maternal blood loss is difficult, those with a past history of abruption, postpartum hemorrhage (blood loss in the first 24 hours after delivery of at least 500 ml and more importantly >1 litre), placenta previa, heritable or acquired coagulation defects (e.g. carriage of hemophilia, von Willebrand's disease, those receiving anticoagulation or with pre-existing DIC due to hemolysis, elevated liver enzymes, and low platelets (HELLP) syndrome or pre-eclampsia), as well as those with complicated or prolonged deliveries, are at increased risk (Table 2.6).

Table 2.6 – Risk of massive obstetric hemorrhage

Complicates 1 in 1000 deliveries	
Maternal death: 1 in 100 000 in developed and 1 in 1000 in developing countries	
Abruptio placenta: fetal mortality <30%	
Placenta previa: fetal mortality <5%	
Loss of 15 000ml, or >25% blood volume, indicates massive loss is likely	
High risk	PMH Abruptio placenta
	PMH PPH
	Hemophilia carriage
	von Willebrand's disease (vWD)
	Heparin
	DIC
	HELLP/PET
Therapy	Crystalloid/colloid
	Red cells
	Early obstetric intervention
	Fluid warmer
	Maintain the PCV/platelets $>50 \times 10^9/l$
	1.5 × blood volume: consider platelet therapy

DIC, Disseminated intravascular coagulation; HELLP, Hemolysis, elevated liver enzymes, and low platelets; PCV, Packed cell volume; PET, Pre-eclampsia; PMH, Past medical history; PPH, Post partum hemorrhage

Massive obstetric hemorrhage remains a major cause of maternal morbidity and mortality, although in recent years the numbers of deaths in the UK have been declining. Such hemorrhage complicates 1 in 1000 deliveries in developed countries and around 1 in 100 000 results in maternal death. Furthermore, in developing countries, maternal death may complicate 1 in 1000 of such events. In approximately half of all women presenting with bleeding from the genital tract after 24 weeks gestation, a diagnosis of placental abruption or placenta previa will be made; no firm diagnosis will be made in the other half, although most may be due to incidental causes such as cervical ectropion. When the blood loss is caused by placental abruption, the fetal mortality is substantial and may complicate up to 30% of cases. When it is due to a placenta previa, the fetal death rate is still considerable at around 5% of cases.

Placental abruption

Placental abruption, or retroplacental hemorrhage, is the premature separation of a normally implanted placenta from the uterine wall, resulting in hemorrhage before the delivery of the fetus. It occurs in around 1 in 80 deliveries. Although maternal mortality is rare, maternal morbidity from hemorrhage, shock, disseminated intravascular coagulation and renal failure is not uncommon. The risk to the fetus depends on the severity of the abruption, the gestation, the birthweight and the amount of concealed hemorrhage. The perinatal mortality with placental abruption is high, and may be >300/1000.

The bleeding, however, may be in whole, or in part, concealed if the hematoma does not reach the margin of the placenta so that the blood loss is revealed. In view of this, the amount of revealed blood loss reflects poorly the degree of hemorrhage, as an enlarged hematoma may be concealed within the uterus. The hematoma may also result in bleeding into the amniotic cavity, with subsequent blood-stained liquor being noted when the membranes rupture. Furthermore, the bleeding may infiltrate the myometrium resulting in so-called Couvelaire uterus. This infiltration of blood into the myometrium is associated with sustained uterine contraction, making the uterus feel 'solid' on examination, provoking labor and reducing utero-placental blood flow with serious compromise to the fetus. Placental abruption may occur at any stage of pregnancy. In severe abruption there may be heavy vaginal bleeding, or increasing abdominal circumference if the bleeding is concealed and retained within the uterus. The woman is usually in severe pain and may be in hypovolemic shock. The uterus may be tender and irritable, with palpable contractions or uterine hypertonus, often resulting in labor. Fetal distress or intrauterine fetal death may be present. In less severe cases, the diagnosis of placental abruption may not be obvious, particularly if the hemorrhage is largely concealed, and such cases may be misdiagnosed as idiopathic preterm labor. Thus, abruption should be considered in any patient presenting with unexplained vaginal bleeding or possible preterm labor, particularly if fetal distress is present.

Placental abruption is a common cause of coagulation failure in pregnancy, and the degree of coagulation disturbance tends to correlate with size of abruption and blood loss. Absence of clotting in the blood within the vagina may be apparent, or there may be bleeding from venepuncture sites or hematuria. FMH may occur and can result in severe fetal anemia or fetal death. If the patient is RhD negative, a Kleihauer (FMH) assessment should be performed, to estimate the volume of FMH in order to provide sufficient anti-RhD immunoglobulin.

Management of massive blood loss

Both clinical assessment and blood pressure measurements are unreliable in estimating the amount of blood loss, and fluid replacement should be guided by other means. Central venous pressure monitoring is essential in serious hemorrhage, although central catheter placement may require correction of coagulopa-

Table 2.7 – Management of massive obstetric hemorrhage

Summon staff (obstetrician, midwife, anesthetist, porter)
Inform (blood transfusion and hematology)
Access (<2 peripheral venous cannulae, chorionic villus sampling (CVP) – if possible, arterial line advised)
Samples (cross-match ≥6 units, coagulation screen, full blood count)
Plasma expanders (hemacel, albumin)
Consider need for uncross-matched blood (O RhD negative – pressure cuff, blood warmer – if possible)
Monitor (blood pressure, pulse, electrocardiogram, blood gas)
Monitor (hemoglobin, platelets, coagulation – including fibrinogen)
Replace (coagulation factors with fresh frozen plasma (FFP)/cryoprecipitate)
Early intervention (artery ligation, Cesarean hysterectomy)
Assess (need for intensive therapy unit)

thy. The immediate concern in the hemorrhaging patient is inadequate circulation and priority should be given to restoring the circulating volume. Large-bore cannulae should be sited, and blood-warming devices and pressure infusion bags should be readily available (Table 2.7).

Blood products are not required for the immediate restoration of the circulating volume, and administration of crystalloid or colloid solutions may be valuable. The crystalloid solutions that may be given include normal saline or Hartmann's solution, but non-salt crystalloids such as 5% dextrose are ineffective. Large doses of colloids, such as gelatin, remain in the circulation longer, an advantage if blood or blood components are not readily available, but a disadvantage if fluid overload and pulmonary edema develop. Dextrans are contraindicated in obstetric hemorrhage since they interfere with platelet function in vivo and blood cross-matching in vitro, and carry a risk of allergic reaction and uterine hypertonus. In all cases, uncross-matched group O, RhD-negative blood should be available within 10 minutes and guidelines suggest that specific cross-matched blood should be available within 30 minutes. In practice group specific blood should be available in 20 minutes, but cross-matched blood may require 40 minutes. The packed cell volume should be maintained at >30 to prevent platelet dysfunction and rapid transfusion should be by means of a fluid warmer (although transfusion should not be delayed if this is not available). Co-infusion of other solutions in the same intravenous access must be avoided, as this will result in red cell lysis. Dilutional thrombocytopenia is likely when 1.5 times the maternal blood volume has been transfused. Where RhD-positive platelets are given to RhD-negative women, there is a requirement to give an appropriate dose of anti-RhD prophylaxis.

Massive blood loss at delivery is rapidly complicated by the development of DIC (see Chapter 8). This may be exacerbated by the hemodilution consequent upon red cell and fluid replacement. In diagnosing DIC, it should be remembered that the maternal plasma fibrinogen is often 4g/l (or more) in normal women at term and that there may be foreshortening of the activated partial thromboplastin time (APTT: usually no more than a decrease in the mean APTT of 4 seconds) with increasing gestation. The level of fibrinogen required for hemostasis should be at least the same as that of non-pregnant subjects at >1.0g/l, using either cryoprecipitate or, if available, a double-virally inactivated fibrinogen concentrate. The platelet count should also be maintained above $50 \times 10^9/l$ when bleeding is continuing, and may need to be $>80 \times 10^9/l$ when an operative intervention is required.

Early intervention to treat the underlying cause is essential with, in particular, rapid delivery in cases of placental abruption or placenta previa. In postpartum hemorrhage associated with uterine atony, rapid treatment with oxytocin or carboprost (a prostaglandin analog) and exclusion of retained placental tissue is required. Further therapy with uterine packing, arterial embolization or hysterectomy may also be required.

CHAPTER 3

Maternal anemia and hemato-oncology in pregnancy

Anemia in pregnancy

A fall in hemoglobin levels with increasing gestation occurs physiologically in pregnancy as a result of hemodilution (see Chapter 1). However, this is distinct from the development of significant anemia, which increases the risk of pregnancy complications. Anemia most commonly develops because of hematinic deficiency, but may also develop in the context of a new red cell or marrow disorder, or because of a pre-existing condition affecting red cell production or survival (see Chapter 9).

As outlined in Chapter 1, a relative reduction in the hematocrit is evident, especially in the first and second trimesters. This leads to a fall in the hemoglobin concentration, which is seen from around 16 weeks gestation until the middle of the third trimester. In subjects with no evidence of iron deficiency this fall is often no more than 1g/dl and results in a normochromic normocytic picture with a hemoglobin concentration of not <11g/dl in the first trimester, or 10g/dl in the second and third trimesters (Table 3.1).

Iron deficiency

Iron has a wide distribution in the body, with around 70% located in hemoglobin and myoglobin. Most non-heme iron is found in ferritin or hemosiderin, in either hepatocytes or macrophages. There is a small amount of iron associated

Table 3.1 – FBC changes in normal pregnancy

NNA from 16 to 34 weeks
Hemoglobin fall <1g/dl
Hemoglobin >11 g/dl in first trimester
Hemoglobin >10 g/dl in third trimester

FBC, Full blood count; NNA, Normochromic normocytic anemia

with the iron-transport protein transferrin; and iron is also required for the function of enzymes, such as catalases and peroxidases. When iron is required for incorporation into these proteins, it is most often derived from recycled iron that has been released from red cell breakdown.

Iron absorption takes place in the first part of the duodenum, and iron balance is achieved by the regulation of this absorption. Iron is absorbed from heme, or from ferrous (non-heme) iron by two distinct pathways. Non-heme iron absorption can be enhanced by ascorbic acid, which assists in the conversion of ferric iron to the ferrous form (the state that is required for absorption). By contrast, phytates (found in cereals) bind non-heme iron and inhibit its absorption, and dietary phosphates also inhibit iron absorption from eggs and milk.

Iron is released from heme on the cell border, and inside the mucosal cell is added to the pool of absorbed iron. Some of the iron is transported into the plasma within a few hours of absorption, but much remains within the mucosal cell. Loss of the mucosal cell (and its iron), by sloughing, appears to have a major role in the regulation of iron balance.

It is likely that iron is transported from the mucosal cell by the action of a transmembrane protein, whose mRNA synthesis is stimulated by iron deficiency. Iron leaving the cell must be oxidized to the ferric state to allow binding to the transport plasma protein (apo-) transferrin. Iron absorption is increased when body iron stores are depleted and reduced when excessive body iron is present. Iron absorption is also increased when there is an increase in erythropoiesis, hypoxia or inflammation. Iron is then transported in the plasma by the glycoprotein transferrin. This is synthesized predominantly in the liver in response to iron deficiency: the total amount of iron that the available plasma transferrin can bind is called the total iron binding capacity (TIBC). In normal non-pregnant subjects around one third of the TIBC is used. Transferrin carries iron to specific transferrin receptors, which are prominent on the developing red cell but are lost as the red cell nears maturity. When transferrin saturation falls to <16% there is insufficient iron delivery to the bone marrow. This results in an increase in free red-cell-derived protophorphyrin, due to the lack of iron leading to a reduction of the incorporation of protophorphyrin into heme. As there is a reduction in the red cell hemoglobin, the red cell continues to divide, resulting in smaller red cells (i.e. microcytosis). Iron deficiency also results in a degree of ineffective erythropoiesis, which results in a reduced red cell half-life (Table 3.2).

Iron deficiency in pregnancy

Pregnancy results in an average loss of maternal iron of around 700mg, associated with the needs of the developing fetus and placenta, as well as the blood loss at delivery. In addition, there is a requirement for around 450mg of iron to support the increase in red cell mass associated with normal pregnancy. Although there is an increase in absorption in the second and third trimesters, there is an iron intake requirement of around 2.5mg/day throughout pregnancy, with perhaps

Table 3.2 – Detection of iron deficiency

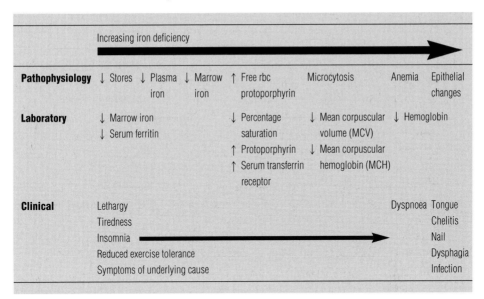

	Increasing iron deficiency →						
Pathophysiology	↓ Stores	↓ Plasma iron	↓ Marrow iron	↑ Free rbc protoporphyrin	Microcytosis	Anemia	Epithelial changes
Laboratory	↓ Marrow iron ↓ Serum ferritin			↓ Percentage saturation ↑ Protoporphyrin ↑ Serum transferrin receptor	↓ Mean corpuscular volume (MCV) ↓ Mean corpuscular hemoglobin (MCH)	↓ Hemoglobin	
Clinical	Lethargy Tiredness Insomnia → Reduced exercise tolerance Symptoms of underlying cause					Dyspnoea	Tongue Chelitis Nail Dysphagia Infection

rbc, Red blood cell

3.0–7.5mg/day required in the third trimester. The support of lactation requires <1mg/day, which is offset by the suppression of menstruation during lactation.

The effect of iron deficiency (prior to the development of anemia) on maternal and fetal wellbeing is not fully understood. There has been speculation that maternal iron deficiency may itself lead to increased blood loss at delivery because of poor myometrial function, although this is by no means proven.

The fetus is 'parasitic' in its acquisition of iron from the mother, but there is the potential that iron deficiency in the mother could result in poor fetal iron stores at delivery, which may have a consequence on early childhood development and behavior (especially if there is subsequent poor iron intake). Iron deficiency has also been implicated in fetal programing, with an increased placental:fetal weight ratio (relative placentomegaly) reported. This, in turn, may also have an influence on maternal blood pressure, and perhaps even the blood pressure of the child when it reaches adulthood. Severe maternal iron deficiency has been associated with premature delivery and low birthweight, but this could also relate to the underlying cause of the maternal anemia. Although repletion of iron leads to an increase in hemoglobin and hematocrit, it may not be associated with any improvement in pregnancy outcome. On account of this, both the importance of iron deficiency and the benefits of iron replacement remain controversial.

Diagnosis of iron deficiency in pregnancy

The signs and symptoms of iron deficiency before the development of anemia are non-specific, and include tiredness and reduced exercise tolerance. There may also be symptoms and signs associated with the underlying cause. Severe iron deficiency anemia (IDA) is associated with atrophy of the papillae, a painful tongue, angular chelitis, nail ridging and, when severe, spooning and (with the development of a post-cricoid web) dysphagia. There may also be an increased risk of infection due to the effect of iron deficiency on cellular immunity and phagocytosis. These changes, however, are extreme and are unlikely to be seen in iron-deficient pregnancies in developed countries. Common causes of iron deficiency in women of childbearing age are shown (Table 3.3).

As noted above, the physiological anemia of pregnancy is associated with a normochromic normocytic picture. It should be noted, however, that a reduction in hemoglobin concentration is a relatively late feature of iron deficiency, and is preceded by depletion in iron stores and serum iron. Furthermore, the reduction in mean corpuscular volume (MCV), which is seen at an early stage with iron deficiency in the non-pregnant, is not so reliable in pregnancy because of the physiological changes in red cell mass and plasma volume. In particular, there may be a rise in the MCV and, thus, a normal MCV does not exclude iron deficiency. In pregnancy the initial appearance of IDA may therefore be normochromic and normocytic, and when there is a hypochromic microcytic picture, the possibility of thalassemia should be considered and excluded.

Although serum ferritin contains little iron, its circulating concentration correlates well with body iron stores, but the use of ferritin to detect iron deficiency may be complicated, as it is an acute phase protein and the lower limit of the reference range is increased in the presence of inflammatory disorders. However, in early pregnancy, reduced serum ferritin concentrations usually provide a reliable indication of iron deficiency, but hemodilution in the second and third trimesters of pregnancy reduces the concentrations of all measures of iron status, and thus the ranges used in non-pregnant women are not always reliable. Nonetheless, a low result still indicates iron deficiency in most pregnant subjects.

Table 3.3 – Causes of iron deficiency

Dietary	Vegetarian/vegan
Blood loss	Menorrhagia
	Peptic ulceration
	Inflammatory bowel disease
	Hemorrhoids
	Varices
	Aspirin
	Anticoagulants
	von Willebrand's disease (vWD)
Malabsorption	Celiac
	Gastrectomy

With regard to other tests of iron deficiency, normal pregnancy (as noted in Chapter 1) is associated with a progressive fall in serum iron, and an increase in both serum TIBC and free protoporphyrin levels. Serum transferrin receptor levels may also increase with gestational age (especially after 20 weeks gestation), and may not fall in response to iron given at a supplemental dose. As noted above, it appears most likely that any increase in serum transferrin receptor levels in later pregnancy relates to increased maternal erythropoiesis. From this it is difficult to know how reliable serum transferrin receptors are in diagnosing IDA in pregnancy. Thus, a combination of assessments should be used to assess iron status when the diagnosis is not clear cut.

Prevention of iron deficiency in pregnancy

The usual practice is to use the hemoglobin concentration as a screening test for iron deficiency, with an assessment at booking and a further one in the early third trimester. Whether routine supplementation to all women is warranted is not resolved, as it is not clear (at least in developed countries) whether the fetus benefits from routine maternal iron prophylaxis (see above). If required, supplementation can be achieved with 60mg of iron/day and 400μg of folic acid given for 6 months of pregnancy (where the prevalence of anemia is low), or continued to include the puerperium (in countries where there is a high incidence of maternal anemia). In the USA, the American College of Obstetricians recommends 30mg of elemental iron/day in the second and third trimesters to all women, irrespective of iron status. This may be a reasonable strategy, as the main side effects from iron are seen at replacement (200mg/day) rather than prophylactic doses, and iron supplementation is safe, as it will not produce a supranormal hemoglobin or hematocrit. There is, however, a consideration that 2–5 in 1000 subjects of European descent may be homozygous (or compound heterozygous) for genes leading to iron overloading and hemochromatosis. Whether iron supplementation in pregnancy in this group results in clinical disease is not clear, as women (perhaps associated with menstrual iron loss) are at a lower risk of organ damage in the reproductive years than men.

Treatment of iron deficiency in pregnancy

The treatment of established iron deficiency is with 200mg/day of elemental iron. In pregnancy, there is no value in using 200mg three times per day, as is often prescribed, as this will only increase the risk of side effects without enhancing the resolution of the anemia. Iron supplements may be associated with gastrointestinal (GI) upset (nausea, heartburn and diarrhea), but this can be dose related and so is usually ameliorated by either a change in the type of oral preparation, or by a reduction in the dose to 100mg/day. In non-pregnant subjects, 200mg/day of ferrous sulphate is expected to result in a rise in hemoglobin of around 1g/dl per week. However, there may be an improvement in wellbeing in advance of any change in the red cell indices, which may reflect improvements in the intracellular metabolic processes where iron is required.

Iron therapy may fail to replete iron stores when there is malabsorption, or when iron lost in bleeding exceeds intake. Occasionally, no improvement is seen, as the diagnosis of iron deficiency is incorrect. However, in the vast majority of instances, failure to improve iron status results from poor compliance with the iron therapy. Vitamin C can enhance absorption of ferrous iron, and this can be achieved by taking the iron supplement with a glass of fresh orange juice or a 50mg tablet of ascorbic acid. It is the authors' practice to routinely prescribe vitamin C with iron supplements for treatment of IDA in pregnancy. For women who have difficulty with swallowing tablets, liquid preparations are available, but these can cause staining of the teeth.

There are a number of forms of parenteral iron therapy, which can be given as a total dose intravenously (iron dextran and iron sucrose compounds) or, in some instances (iron dextran), as multiple doses intramuscularly. The indications for parenteral therapy include malabsorption and failure of compliance with oral therapy, and there may also be requirement when erythropoietin is being used.

With the exception of renal failure requiring dialysis or malabsorption, parenteral iron probably does not produce a faster hemoglobin response than oral iron. Despite this, parenteral iron therapy is often used when severe IDA is diagnosed at an advanced stage in pregnancy.

With intravenous dextran (and to some extent iron sucrose) compounds there is a small risk of an anaphylactoid reaction (estimated at around 0.6% of recipients), and it is recommended that a test dose of 25mg of iron should be given over 15 minutes before a therapeutic dose is given. With intramuscular preparations there is a risk of pain or abscess formation, skin pigmentation and local sarcoma at the injection site. Overall, some side effects are reported in around 25% of subjects receiving parenteral iron therapy. The majority of these are mild, and include headache, urticaria and nausea, but serious adverse events have been reported to occur in as many as 5% of subjects. In around 1% of recipients of either preparation there is also the possibility of a delayed reaction with myalgia, arthralgia, lymphadenopathy and fever.

Folic acid deficiency

Folates are found in a wide variety of foodstuffs, but liver, green vegetables (such as brocolli, asparagus, sprouts and spinach), mushrooms and nuts contain the highest quantities. Cooking, however, may result in a substantial loss in the folic acid available from such produce. The average daily requirement in non-pregnant subjects is around 100μg/day, with an average Western diet supplying around 250μg/day. Folic acid is predominantly absorbed in the upper small intestine, with 50–90% of food folates presented to the upper small bowel being absorbed. Folic acid and its metabolites are lost in the urine, through the skin and there is also an enterohepatic circulation through the bile. Folic acid deficiency is most commonly due to dietary insufficiency associated with alcoholism and poverty. Malabsorption, due to gluten-induced enteropathy, partial gastrectomy or Crohn's disease may also exacerbate dietary insufficiency, and such patients should routinely receive folate supplements throughout their pregnancy. Other subjects at risk include those with an increased usage of folate. This includes those with chronic hemolytic conditions (e.g. hemoglobinopathy, sickle-cell syndromes, red cell membrane and enzyme disorders, myeloproliferative disorders, and autoimmune hemolytic anemia), those taking antiepileptic drugs (e.g. carbamazepine), and those requiring dialysis (where there may be an increase in loss through dialysis due to loose plasma protein binding) (Table 3.4).

Polyglutamated folate is an essential coenzyme in the transfer of single carbon units required for the manufacture of DNA and RNA. By this, and other means, folic acid may function to reduce oxidative potential. Folic acid, along with vitamin B_{12} and vitamin B_6, assists in the homocysteine (HCY)–methionine pathway (Figure 3.1), where the presence of folic acid drives the production of methionine from HCY, leading to a reduction in the plasma levels of HCY.

Circulating HCY is readily oxidized, and as a result may increase the generation of superoxide (O_2^-) and hydrogen peroxide (H_2O_2) species. These free radicals can induce oxidation of low-density lipoproteins (LDL) in the endothelium, and it has been proposed that prolonged exposure of the endothelium to HCY results in exhaustion of the mechanisms of endothelial protection against HCY. HCY also has an effect on a number of aspects of coagulation, which includes upregulation of Factor (F) V generation and downregulation of the anticoagulants activated protein C (aPC) and thrombomodulin.

Although most subjects are diagnosed with deficiency because of an incidental finding of a raised MCV, folate and vitamin B_{12} deficiency may present with

Table 3.4 – Cause of folic acid deficiency

Dietary	Alcoholism
	Poverty
	Adolescence
Malabsorption	Gluten-induced enteropathy (celiac)
Increased use	Chronic hemolysis
	Congenital red cell disorders
	Hemoglobinopathy
	Myeloproliferative disorders
Loss	Dialysis
Miscellaneous	Anticonvulsants

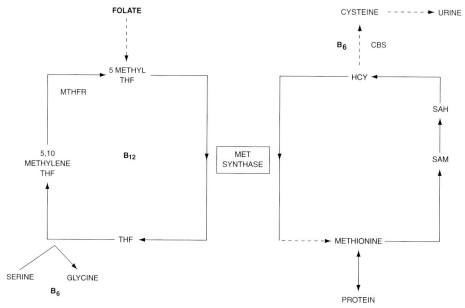

Figure 3.1 Homocysteine (HCY)–methionine pathway
Methionine is converted to S-adenosyl methionine (SAM); this is converted via S-adenosyl homocysteine (SAH) to HCY. HCY is converted via cystathionine beta-synthase (CBS) to cysteine, which requires vitamin B_6 (B_6) as a cofactor; cysteine is excreted in the urine. HCY leads to the reformation of methionine, via methionine synthase (MET SYNTHASE); this requires folate and vitamin B_{12} (B_{12}) and methylene tetrahydrofolate reductase (MTHFR).

anemia (Table 3.5). Non-specific symptoms such as lethargy, breathlessness and, occasionally, anginal symptoms may be accompanied by other features such as GI upset, angular cheilitis and glossitis. In more severe cases there may be jaundice (due to a rise in unconjugated bilirubin from ineffective erythropoiesis), and a reduction in both white cell and platelet production, leading to infection and bruising. The effect on platelets and leukocytes is often forgotten and clinicians should be aware that incidental findings of thrombocytopenia on a blood film may reflect folate deficiency.

Table 3.5 – Common causes of macrocytosis

Vitamin B_{12} deficiency
Folate deficiency
Alcohol
Hypothyroidism
Pregnancy
Liver disease
Myelodysplasia
Hemolysis

Folic acid deficiency in pregnancy

In pregnancy folic acid requirements increase to around 400µg/day, due to the demands of the developing fetus and increased folate catabolism, which is accompanied by a gradual fall in serum folate levels with increasing gestation. Those with an inadequate dietary intake are at risk of the development of a macrocytic anemia. The prevalence of deficiency is <5% of subjects in developed countries and may be as low as 0.5% where there are routine prophylaxis programs. Folate deficiency is more common in multiple pregnancy, frequent childbirth and when the mother is still an adolescent. In the first trimester, folic acid deficiency may not often present with anemia but, linked with HCY generation, is associated with fetal neural tube defects. Folate deficiency anemia often coexists with iron deficiency (due to a generally poor diet), and more often presents at the end of pregnancy or in the early puerperium. Very occasionally, and often in the presence of infection, folate deficiency may present as an acute aplasia (with pancytopenia accompanied by megaloblastic erythropoiesis in the bone marrow), or come to light as a result of thrombocytopenia.

Diagnosis of folic acid deficiency in pregnancy

The diagnosis of megaloblastic anemia in pregnancy is suggested by the presence of a macrocytic blood picture (MCV >100fl), the presence of right-shifted neutrophils (>5 segments) on the blood film and, in severe cases, a mild leukopenia and thrombocytopenia (platelets $50–100 \times 10^9$/l). A reduction in serum folate levels is a sensitive test of folic acid deficiency; however, it may also be reduced if there has been only a recent folate lack in the diet and also reduces with increasing gestation. Falsely normal serum folate results may also be seen in acute liver failure, renal failure and vitamin B_{12} deficiency. Measurement of red cell folate is more representative of body stores and is less affected by recent changes in dietary intake, but can be falsely normal if there has been a recent red cell transfusion, and has been reported to occasionally rise in an otherwise normal pregnancy (Table 3.6).

In detecting folate deficiency in pregnancy there may diagnostic difficulties, as macrocytosis can be seen in pregnant subjects without megaloblastosis, and is also seen in subjects with alcohol excess, hemolysis, hypothyroidism, vitamin B_{12} deficiency, or renal failure. If, in such circumstances, folate assays are not clear-cut, megalobastic erythropoiesis can be demonstrated by bone marrow examination. The principal feature of megaloblastosis is asynchrony of cytoplasmic and nuclear development of red cell precursors (i.e. an immature nuclear appearance with mature hemoglobinised cytoplasm). The diagnosis can be complicated when there is also iron deficiency, as the MCV may be normal. Usually, however, the blood film is dimorphic (i.e. showing evidence of both the microcytes of iron deficiency and the macrocytes of megaloblastic erythropoiesis).

Table 3.6 – Source of Hematinics

Hematinic	Source	Pregnancy requirement	Measure	Measure limitations	Pregnancy prophylaxis	Deficiency treatment
Vitamin B$_{12}$	Animals	3µg/day	Serum vitamin B$_{12}$ Urinary methyl-malonic acid (MMA)	Gestation effect Poor correlation with vitamin B$_{12}$	?3µg/day	1mg
Folate	Vegetables, liver, nuts	400µg/day	Mean corpuscular volume (MCV) Serum folate rbc folate Homocysteine (HCY)	Gestation effect or iron deficiency anemia (IDA) Recent diet/renal/ vitamin B$_{12}$ deficiency Transfusion Poor correlation with folate	400µg/day to 5mg/day	15mg/day
Iron	Meat, vegetables dairy	2.5mg/day to 3.0–7.5mg/day	MCV Ferritin Iron/total iron binding capacity (TIBC) Serum transferrin (sTF) receptors Marrow	Gestation effect or thalassemia Acute phase reactant and gestation effect Gestation effect Gestation effect Pain	30–60µg/day	200mg/day

rbc, Red blood cell

Prophylaxis and treatment of folic acid deficiency in pregnancy

Given the potential for mild folate deficiency to be associated with neural tube defects, folic acid supplementation is routinely given in the first trimester at a dose of 400µg/day. This also extends to those planning pregnancy with a recommendation that such supplements be taken for 3 months prior to conception. This routine prophylaxis results in at least a 70% reduction in the risk of neural tube defects. There may also be potential benefits to other pregnancy complications, such as pre-eclampsia and intrauterine growth restriction, where hyperhomocysteinemia may be a pathophysiological factor. Folic acid will reduce HCY concentrations, but whether prolonged prophylaxis is effective in preventing or amelioratiiong these problems is not yet established. At any rate, there has been no suggestion that such prolonged prophylaxis, at a dose of 400µg/day, is detrimental to the mother or fetus. In those who have had a previous child affected by a neural tube defect, folic acid therapy (at a dose of at least 5mg/day) should be given when pregnancy is planned and for the first trimester. As noted above, prophylaxis is also required for subjects with chronic inherited or acquired red cell disorders. In some such cases, there may also be a role for adding iron prophylaxis.

Proven folic acid deficiency anemia should be treated with folic acid therapy at a dose of 5mg×3/day. In all such cases of anemia, vitamin B_{12} deficiency must also be excluded, as folate supplementation may improve the anemia of vitamin B_{12} deficiency but exacerbate the neurological deterioration associated with it (see below). In general, it is also good practice to check the vitamin B_{12} status of all those presenting with significant folic acid deficiency. Folinic acid – a form of folic acid which can bypass a block in the methylene tetrahydrofolate reductase enzyme induced by methotrexate, or an excess dose of trimethoprim – can be used to reverse folate inhibitory drugs, and is occasionally used when there is severe folate deficient anemia from other causes.

In all women with evidence of folic acid deficiency it is important to take a dietary history, and if the diet is lacking in folate-rich foods to provide dietary advice.

Vitamin B_{12} deficiency

As shown in Figure 3.1, vitamin B_{12} is another essential cofactor in both the manufacture of DNA and the disposal of HCY. Vitamin B_{12} is also essential in the conversion of methylmalonyl-CoA to succinyl-CoA. In addition to similar symptoms of anemia to those observed with folate deficiency, vitamin B_{12} deficiency also results in a demyelinating neuropathy affecting the pyramidal and posterior tracts of the spinal cord, the peripheral nerves and the optic tract.

Vitamin B_{12} is only synthesized by microorganisms and the only source available to humans is derived from animal foodstuffs. Of these, liver, kidney, meat, fish, chicken and dairy products are the most important sources. Thus vegetarians, and particularly vegans, are most at risk of nutritional deficiency. Unlike dietary folates, cooking does not destroy vitamin B_{12}. On average, there is a body store of around 3mg, with a daily dietary requirement of around 3μg/day. As a result, it may take 3–5 years after the onset of a dietary lack for clinical deficiency to become apparent.

A very small amount of vitamin B_{12} is absorbed passively in the duodenum and ileum, but the major site of absorption is by a specific mechanism in the ileum, requiring the combination of vitamin B_{12} and intrinsic factor (produced in the gastric parietal cells). There is also an enterohepatic circulation of up to 5μg of vitamin B_{12}, which is the reabsorbed in the terminal ileum.

The causes of vitamin B_{12} deficiency include a dietary lack, which is most often seen in vegans who do not eat animal products. In addition to dietary deficiency, other causes include pernicious anemia (due to a defect of intrinsic factor production), partial gastric resection, ileal resection, intestinal stagnant loop syndrome, Crohn's disease, tapeworms and tropical sprue. In addition, deficiency of folate can result in small bowel malabsorption of vitamin B_{12}.

As noted above, vitamin B_{12} deficiency should be excluded in all cases of megaloblastic anemia, by assessment of serum vitamin B_{12} levels. Occasionally, low levels, associated with neurological disturbance, can be seen even in the absence of anemia.

In non-pregnant subjects, a diagnosis of pernicious anemia (PA) can be made by demonstrating a lack of intrinsic factor secretion using vitamin B_{12} binding studies (demonstrating the effect on urinary vitamin B_{12} excretion of adding intrinsic factor to an oral dose of radiolabelled vitamin B_{12}). Malabsorption is indicated by a low urinary response to the radiolabelled oral vitamin B_{12} dose, that is not sufficiently improved by the addition of intrinsic factor. Such a result may require other intestinal absorption studies and bowel imaging to reach a diagnosis.

In pregnancy, other tests, such as those to detect antibodies to intrinsic factor or parietal cells, are useful to confirm the diagnosis of PA. Of these, intrinsic factor antibodies (although seen in other autoimmune conditions) are more specific than parietal cell antibodies for pernicious anemia. Indeed, such antibodies have been shown to cross the placenta and to lead to intrinsic factor deficiency in the newborn.

The diagnosis of vitamin B_{12} deficiency can be confirmed by a therapeutic trial of parenteral vitamin B_{12} (which will happen incidentally in non-pregnant subjects when vitamin B_{12} binding studies are performed, as a non-radiolabelled parenteral vitamin B_{12} injection is required to complete the study). After such a trial, a reticulocyte response should be evident between 3 and 7 days. As there may be difficulty in interpreting borderline vitamin B_{12} levels, other assessments to demonstrate tissue deficiency, such as plasma HCY levels (which correlate well with folate but not with vitamin B_{12}) and the urinary methylmalonic acid (MMA):creatinine ratio (which can be determined by a single urinary measure), have been proposed. The level of serum MMA, however, is less sensitive and specific than urinary estimates, as it is also raised in renal insufficiency, thyroid disease, pregnancy and when there is dehydration.

Vitamin B_{12} deficiency in pregnancy

Vitamin B_{12} levels may fall by 30–50% during pregnancy, with evidence of reduced levels in the first trimester in some individuals. This occurs despite a diet adequate in vitamin B_{12}, and is likely to be due to a combination of increasing maternal plasma volume, hormonal changes, increasing maternal requirement and transfer to the fetus. It appears that there is a poor correlation between maternal serum vitamin B_{12} and serum HCY levels in pregnancy, and, in non-anemic pregnant subjects, no correlation between urinary MMA levels and serum vitamin B_{12} has been reported. This suggests that the physiological reduction in serum vitamin B_{12} in pregnancy does not represent a true tissue deficiency.

A correlation between maternal and neonatal vitamin B_{12} levels has, however, been reported. Thus, although mild vitamin B_{12} deficiency appears compatible with a normal pregnancy outcome, it could result in a low level of vitamin B_{12} in the offspring (particularly if the baby is subsequently breastfed). Lower levels of vitamin B_{12} have also been found in women who have had a child with a neural tube defect and in those with early recurrent abortions. Indeed, it is thought that persisting vitamin B_{12} deficiency can result in infertility, but the role of lesser deficiency in fetal cognitive development or birthweight is not yet resolved. In countries where a vegetarian diet is the norm, folate deficiency is less common and vitamin B_{12} deficiency may play a more important role in the development of neural tube defects.

Autoimmune hemolytic anemia (AIHA)

On average, red cells survive for 120 days in the circulation. If an autoantibody develops which can result in red cell lysis, the destruction occurs either within the circulation and/or within the liver and spleen. Such autoantibodies may be of IgG, IgM or IgA class, and this phenomenon is often classified, by the temperature range of the antibody, into cold or warm acting.

In general, warm antibodies have their maximal effect at $37°C$ and cold-acting ones have increasing activity with decreasing body temperature. Warm antibodies are typically: of IgG type; may or may not result in complement binding to the red cells; and most often result in loss of red cells in the spleen or liver. Cold antibodies are: most often of IgM type; and are often capable of fixing complement and leading to intravascular hemolysis. There are, of course, exceptions to this and AIHA can be associated with a mixed antibody pattern.

The mechanism whereby these antibodies develop is essentially unknown, but may be related to a genetic predisposition through the patient's human leukocyte antigen (HLA) type, molecular mimicry (where there is a similarity to a microorganism) and/or involve a change in immune tolerance.

Red cell destruction leads to an increase in red cell production in the bone marrow (erythroid hyperplasia), with the release of early cells (called reticulocytes) into the peripheral circulation (Table 3.7). Reticulocytes, unlike mature

Table 3.7 – Diagnosis of Intravascular Hemolysis

Macrocytosis
Reticulocytosis
Spherocytosis
↓ Serum haptoglobin
↑ Plasma hemoglobin
Hemosiderinuria/hemoglobinuria
↑ Lactate dehydrogenase
Positive direct antiglobulin (Coombs') test

red cells, contain detectable RNA. If there is brisk intravascular breakdown there will be a reduction in the level of the serum protein haptoglobin, which complexes with hemoglobin to remove it from the circulation. There may also be detectable plasma hemoglobin and evidence of hemoglobinuria. When hemolysis is less marked, free hemoglobin is catabolized by the renal tubular cells to hemosiderin, which is detectable in the urine. The enzyme lactate dehydrogenase is also released from damaged red cells and the hemoglobin metabolite bilirubin is released from the reticulo-endothelial system to be conjugated in the liver and excreted in bile into the gut. This fecal urobilinogen is reabsorbed from the gut into the circulation and is then excreted in the kidneys, and is also detectable in the urine.

The presence of an antibody bound to a red cell antigen can be demonstrated by the direct antiglobulin test (the Coombs' test) if it is IgG. If it is IgM or IgA, its presence can be inferred by a positive antiglobulin test that has detected the presence of complement on the red cell surface. The presence of bound antibody or complement does not itself indicate hemolysis, but simply that an autoantibody is present. Antibody-mediated damage results in the loss of red cell membrane and this leads to the formation of detectable spherocytes within the circulation.

Warm-acting autoantibodies are most often IgG and, although they occasionally have a specificity for RhC, e, Kell or RhD, they most often react equally with a number of donor red cells in cross-matching procedures (see Chapter 2). The consequences of such antibodies can vary from an incidental positive direct antiglobulin test to fulminant hemolysis. The majority of clinically affected subjects present with a chronic stable anemia.

More than 90% of cold antibodies have the *I* red cell antigen as the target, with the remainder aimed at the *i* antigen. In the case of the condition known as paroxysmal cold hemoglobinuria (classically associated with syphilis, but also associated with viral infections), the antibodies are most likely to be of polyclonal IgG type and specific for the *P* red cell antigen. In this disorder the IgG binds in the patient's periphery (at cooler temperatures), but then results in intravascular lysis when it binds complement in the warmer central circulation.

AIHA in pregnancy

In women of childbearing age, cold-acting IgM antibodies are now most often idiopathic, or are found in association with the presence of autoimmune disorders or infections, such as infectious mononucleosis, measles or mumps. If these antibodies are only active at <30°C, they are unlikely to cause significant hemolysis.

Warm antibodies in this age group are often idiopathic, but can also be associated with autoimmune disorders, some therapeutic drugs (classically penicillin, quinidine or methydopa), viral infections, immunodeficiency (including HIV), lymphoproliferative disorders and other malignancies (Table 3.8). The rate of

Table 3.8 – Causes of autoimmune hemolytic anemia (AIHA)

Predominantly cold	Autoimmune disorders
	Infectious mononucleosis
	Measles
	Mumps
	Idiopathic
Predominantly warm	Idiopathic
	Autoimmune disorders
	Drugs
	HIV
	Other viral infections
	Pregnancy
	Lymphoma/malignancy

AIHA in pregnancy appears to be higher than that of subjects of a similar age (1 in 50 000 versus 0.2 in 50 000), with the possibility of increasing hemolysis with increasing gestation and remission after delivery in some cases. As with non-pregnant subjects, there is the possibility of concomitant immune thrombocytopenia (Evan's syndrome). In addition, when there is a maternal IgG antibody, there is the possibility of transplacental passage of the antibody resulting in an asymptomatic positive direct antiglobulin test in the baby, or self-limiting infant hemolysis. In fact, a pregnancy-specific AIHA can occur. This remits after pregnancy but can return in subsequent pregnancies.

Treatment of AIHA

Drug triggers for hemolysis should be sought and any potential implicated drugs excluded, if possible. No treatment is required for asymptomatic direct antiglobulin test positivity. When treatment is required for an idiopathic AIHA, the first-line therapy should be corticosteroids. Most often this is given as oral prednisolone at a dose of 1–2mg/kg body weight. When a stable hemoglobin is achieved, the steroids are reduced at a rate of 5–10mg/week until a maintenance dose is achieved. With high doses, the mother will be at risk of steroid-related side effects, but at maintenance doses this is not usually a problem. However, any mother on steroid supplements should receive 150mg of hydrocortisone 8 hourly at the time of delivery. Fetal problems are not associated with steroid therapy, although with very prolonged use of high doses (>30mg/day of prednisolone), fetal adrenal suppression can occur, and the pediatricians should be alerted to this possibility.

Where steroids cannot be used, or fail, regular infusions of intravenous human normal immunoglobulin may be used to maintain hemoglobin levels. In all cases, folic acid supplementation is required to prevent hemolysis-induced folic acid deficiency. When transfusion is required, the principles detailed in Chapter 2 should be followed. Other therapies such as azathioprine have been used during pregnancy, but splenectomy should be reserved for life-threatening, treatment-resistant anemia whilst the woman is still pregnant.

Hemato-oncology and pregnancy

Although a number of different hematological malignancies do occur in women of childbearing age, it is rare for an acute disorder to be diagnosed for the first time during pregnancy, but it is increasingly likely that someone who has been previously treated for a malignant hematological condition will present for ante-natal care. The specific care of acute hematological malignancy is a rapidly changing area which is beyond the scope of this book, but the general principles of management of malignant hematological conditions that may be found in pregnant subjects will be outlined.

Essential thrombocythemia (ET)

ET is a myeloproliferative disorder, characterized by a persistent elevation in platelet count (i.e. beyond the local reference range), occurring in the absence of iron deficiency, bleeding, malignancy or other myeloproliferative and connective tissue disorders. Although it is a disease of late, middle and old age, an excess of cases around 30 years of age has been reported. In practice, it should be remembered, however, that around 85% of cases of thrombocytosis are reactive rather than a primary phenomenon (Table 3.9).

Bleeding is the most frequent symptom in the majority of ET cases, and in young women the clinical course is most often benign. Subjects are, however, at increased risk of myocardial ischemia, transient neurological dysfunction (characterized by headache, lightheadedness or parasthesia), peripheral arterial occlusion (and erythromelalgia) and venous thrombosis. These complications are more likely in older subjects, although those with a platelet count of $1000–2000 \times$

Table 3.9 – Causes of thrombocytosis

Reactive	85%	Bleeding
		Iron deficiency
		Malignancy
		Connective tissue disorders
		Splenectomy
Primary	15%	Essential thrombocythemia (ET)
		Other myeloproliferative disorders

10^9/l, and especially those with evidence of a platelet function defect (or acquired von Willebrand's disease), may be at particular risk of bleeding. Those with a past history of thrombosis or bleeding should be considered at high risk of another thrombotic or bleeding event. Whether there is any impact of co-inheritance of thrombophilia on the occurrence of thrombosis in ET is unknown.

ET in pregnancy

Although, as noted above, the clinical course of ET is most often benign in the young, there are reports of an association with an adverse pregnancy outcome. The incidence of adverse effects comes predominantly from case reports or small case series. From these, the most common complication is miscarriage (from 25 to 40%), with around a third occurring in the first trimester. The occurrence of late fetal loss may also be increased, with stillbirth/intrauterine death reported to occur in 5–11% of pregnancies, and there may also be an increased risk of growth restriction and pre-term delivery. The consequences to the mother appears more favorable, with the incidence of thrombosis at <3.5%, and most probably less <1%, for significant vascular occlusion (cerebral venous thrombosis or transient cerebral ischemia of arterial origin). The presence of placental thrombosis has been reported in association with late fetal loss and bleeding has been reported in <10% of cases, with the majority of events of a minor nature.

As with normal subjects, pregnancy is associated with a reduction in the platelet count in subjects with ET. Whether the degree of fall in platelet count is related to pregnancy outcome is not clear, and, in general, experience in a previous pregnancy, or the maternal pre-morbid condition, do not clearly indicate the prognosis in the current pregnancy.

A platelet level of $1000-1500 \times 10^9$/l has been suggested as the level at which cytoreduction is required. Despite this, it has been suggested that chemotherapeutic agents can be safely withheld in pregnancy in subjects <30 years of age. At present there is insufficient evidence, however, to recommend that therapy can be safely withheld in asymptomatic individuals when a diagnosis is first made during pregnancy. However, cytoreduction should be avoided in the first trimester if possible.

Hydroxycarbamide (otherwise known as hydroxyurea, a ribonucleotide reductase inhibitor) is widely used in non-pregnant subjects and has been shown to reduce the risk of thrombosis. There is, however, the potential for fetal teratogenicity and its safety in pregnancy, especially in the first trimester, is not known.

Although anagrelide has been used to treat ET, it appears to be less effective in the prevention of thrombotic events and possibly carries an increased risk of myelofibrosis. It therefore has a very limited role in the management of ET generally. As it also crosses the placenta, as well as the breast, and there is limited information on its safety in pregnancy, it should not be used in this circumstance.

In the main, the decision for therapy is an individual one. In those where chemotherapeutic agents are required to achieve cytoreduction, α-interferon may be the drug of choice as it does not cross the placenta, although it can be present in breast milk.

In those subjects taking hydroxycarbamide, when pregnancy is planned, α-interferon should be substituted 3–6 months prior to a planned conception. It has been claimed that α-interferon improves pregnancy outcome in those with a previous poor pregnancy, but this is by no means proven.

The role of platelet-pheresis is poorly defined, as it is not clear whether it influences outcome, but it is well tolerated and may be useful when an acute reduction in platelet numbers is required. However, multiple (often twice weekly) treatments are usually required to sustain a reduction in the platelet count.

Antiplatelet agents may be used to reduce the risk of placental thrombosis and may also assist in the prevention of maternal thrombosis. This may be particularly useful when there are symptoms of microvascular thrombosis, but may exacerbate any platelet defect or acquired von Willebrand's deficiency.

Heparin may be employed as thromboprophylaxis in those subjects with a previous vascular occlusion, but its role in the prolongation of pregnancy is not known. In addition, the necessity and timing of thromboprophylaxis in asymptomatic subjects remains unknown.

Paroxysmal nocturnal hemoglobinuria (PNH)

PNH is rare, but can present in women of childbearing age. It is associated with episodes of intravascular hemolysis resulting in hemoglobinuria as well as anemia, thrombocytopenia and leukopenia (Table 3.10). It is also associated with

Table 3.10 – Paroxysmal nocturnal hemoglobinuria (PNH) features

Intravascular hemolysis
Thrombocytopenia
Leukopenia
Median survival 10–15 years
Thrombosis/bleeding/infection/leukemia/aplasia/remission
↓ GPI anchor → ↓ CD 59 on RBC/PMN
↑ Sensitivity to complement
Washed cellular products for transfusion
Significant fetal and maternal morbidity/mortality

CD, Cluster of differentiation; GPI, Glycophosphortidylinositol; PMN, Polymorphonuclear cell; RBC; Red blood cell an increased risk of venous thrombosis, which classically occurs in the portal or hepatic tracts, and may result in a peripheral deep vein thrombosis. The median survival from diagnosis is 10–15 years, with the potential for fatal thrombosis, thrombocytopenia-associated bleeding or infection. Very occasionally, the condition may present or terminate with aplastic anemia or acute leukemia. There are also reports, however, of spontaneous resolution.

PNH is caused by a clonal defect in the body's own defences against the action of complement. This defence is mediated by a number of proteins that are attached to cell membranes by a glycophosphatidylinositol (GPI) anchor. An acquired mutation in the PIG-A gene on the X chromosome results in defective synthesis of this anchor, with the resultant loss of function of the proteins that should be attached to it.

The disorder was in the past diagnosed by the Ham's acid lysis test, which demonstrates increased red cell lysis by the action of endogenous complement. However, as it is recognized that this mutation affects all cells of the granulocyte line (i.e. red cells, platelets and white cells (excluding lymphocytes)), the diagnosis is now made by demonstrating (using flow cytometry) a significant reduction in one of the GPI-anchored proteins. This is usually achieved by demonstrating a reduction in the expression of the cluster of differentiation (CD) molecule 59 on either the red cell or the neutrophil.

Although there has been a great increase in the understanding of the mechanism of PNH, there has been little advance in its therapy, with allogenic bone marrow transplant being the only curative treatment. The mainstays of routine therapy remain red cell and platelet components, anticoagulation and the treatment of infection.

PNH in pregnancy

The management of PNH in pregnancy requires consideration of a number of aspects of the disease. The thrombotic effect is likely to be due to an interaction between white cells or platelets with complement, but may also, at least in part, be mediated through circulating pro-coagulant microparticles, which are also found in antiphospholipid syndromes. Thus, there may be similar processes and consequences in both disorders.

Therapeutic anticoagulation is needed in those who have previously experienced thrombosis. The role of thromboprophylaxis in those who have not yet had a thrombosis is not known, but we would recommend this in all cases. As with other disorders requiring anticoagulation, this is best achieved in pregnancy with therapeutic or prophylactic dose, low-molecular-weight heparin (LMWH) antepartum, and with warfarin or continued LMWH (avoiding the need for international normalized ratio (INR) monitoring) in the puerperium.

PNH is also associated with thrombocytopenia, and there may be an exaggeration of the normal thrombocytopenia of pregnancy. It has been suggested that the platelet count should be maintained at $>30 \times 10^9/l$ throughout pregnancy.

This may be difficult to achieve and will require washed platelet component therapy to reduce the risk of exposure to exogenous complement. There is little evidence that this is required and in the absence of bleeding problems and with a platelet count >10–20 × 10^9/l, the present authors would manage the patient conservatively. As with other conditions (see Chapter 8), an adequate platelet count is, however, required for delivery or Cesarean section, thus washed platelet preparations are best reserved for delivery.

Epidural analgesia may be problematic from both thrombocytopenia and anti-coagulant viewpoints, and so may be unavailable to such women. In all events, a planned delivery will most often be required to ensure adequate hemostasis. Anemia is common, and also requires the provision of washed red cell components. The development of severe anemia may also have a bearing on fetal oxygenation and development. Following delivery, the combined oral contraceptive must be avoided because of the thrombotic risk.

The maternal mortality may be of the order of 20% in cases of PNH during pregnancy. Pregnancy may be associated with a substantial requirement for maternal platelet and red cell component therapy, and an increased risk of both venous thrombosis and infection. Although successful pregnancies have been reported, the fetal mortality may be as high as 10%, with 50% delivering pre-term, and there is also an increased risk of fetal growth restriction in those mothers with severe anemia.

Acute leukemia in pregnancy

Although relatively rare, acute leukemia may present for the first time in pregnancy. Of those that do, the majority will be acute myeloid leukemia (around 70%), with the remainder of acute lymphoblastic type (Table 3.11). Affected subjects often present with symptoms of anemia or infection. In general, such leukemias have a long-term survival of around 50% and initial remission is likely in around 75%. Without treatment there will be, however, a rapid deterioration, with death frequently occurring within a few months of diagnosis. Overall, the pregnancy has no effect on the leukemia and there is no evidence that a termination will improve the maternal outcome from the disease. The presence of pregnancy may however delay treatment, as there is concern that chemo- or radiotherapies will have a deleterious effect on the fetus. This is most likely to be the case if treatment is administered during the first trimester, when the risk of teratogenesis from acute leukemia therapy has been suggested to be of the order of 20%. It seems unlikely that treatment after the first trimester will lead to significant fetal abnormality, although a transient fetal myelosuppression may be evident after treatment in later pregnancy. Overall, miscarriage, growth restriction and stillbirth is probably higher in affected pregnancies, but whether this results from the maternal condition or the treatment is unknown. In general, a termination is often offered to those mothers presenting in the first trimester. If the pregnancy is continuing, a delay in therapy should be avoided, but may be

Table 3.11 – Leukemia and lymphoma in pregnancy

Acute leukemia	70% of acute leukemias will be AML In this group there is a 40–50% long-term survival Patients present with pancytopenia Chemotherapy in the first trimester may run the risk of teratogenesis (particularly methotrexate) There may be an increased risk of IUGR/stillbirth If the patient has thrombocytopenia, bleeding at delivery is possible
Lymphoma	Hodgkin's disease is probably more likely to present than NHL Hodgkin's disease: treatment delay/modification may be possible NHL: full treatment usually required If chest radiotherapy required then fetal shielding is effective Pregnancy possible if previous radiotherapy to the abdomen, unless it was radical uterine radiotherapy
There may be few late effects on children exposed to chemo- or radiotherapy in utero	

AML, Acute myeloid leukemia; IUGR, Intrauterine growth restriction; NHL, Non-Hodgkin's lymphoma.

contemplated (dependent upon maternal health) until the beginning of the second trimester. In all cases, treatment should be instigated as soon as is practical and methotrexate (a methylene tetrahydrofolate reductase inhibitor used in acute lymphoblastic leukemia treatment) should be avoided, as it may have a profound affect on fetal development. Presentation in the late third trimester may also lead to a delay in treatment being considered until after delivery. In such cases, delivery may have to take account of the risks of maternal hemorrhage and infection, but there are a number of reports of a successful pregnancy outcome in such cases.

Lymphoma in pregnancy

The co-occurrence of lymphoma and pregnancy is relatively rare (Table 3.11). As with the treatment of acute leukemia, management should consider the maternal wishes, the type of disease, the likelihood of cure, the gestation at diagnosis, the possibility of fetal effects and the possibility of collection of ovarian material for storage. In the vast majority of lymphomas there is no evidence that the lymphoma itself influences pregnancy, or that the pregnancy has an adverse influence on the lymphoma.

When Hodgkin's disease presents in the first trimester, a number of options should be considered. Where there is aggressive disease, therapy may be required immediately and the possibility of termination should be discussed. When, as is more common, there is a lower grade of disease there are a number of possible therapeutic options. These include monitoring the disease without therapy, the use of single agent therapy (such as vinblastine) to control the disease until definitive treatment is considered appropriate, use of a modified chemotherapeutic regimen, full therapeutic combinations, or radiotherapy (where appropriate) with fetal shielding. Non-Hodgkin's lymphoma (NHL) usually presents later and often with more aggressive disease. In most cases, immediate standard-dose therapy is required and should not be delayed. However, if either NHL or Hodgkin's disease presents in late pregnancy, there may be scope to withhold treatment until safe delivery can be achieved.

There is no suggestion that diagnostic radiation or nuclear diagnostic tests themselves should be an indication for termination. Indeed supradiaphragmatic irradiation, including spiral computerized tomography (CT) scanning, does not expose the fetus to a significant radiation dose and is considered safe for the fetus. Indeed, despite the caution expressed about chemotherapy (especially when given in the first trimester), long-term follow-up of offspring of those who received treatment for acute leukemia, Hodgkin's disease or NHL, does not show any evidence of an adverse effect on intellectual development, growth or the occurrence of malignancy.

In subjects who have been previously treated for lymphoma there is an increased risk of ovarian failure and premature menopause. This is particularly the case in women treated after the age of 25 years with a combination of chemotherapy and infradiaphragmatic radiotherapy. However, even those who have undergone high-dose regimens may conceive (with hormone replacement) with a successful outcome. Abdominal radiation affecting only a part of the uterus does not preclude pregnancy, but when radiotherapy has involved the uterus, early delivery and growth restriction may occur in subsequent preg-nancies. At present, the significance of these observations is not clear. After radical radiotherapy the uterus is unlikely to support conception, even if there is satisfactory ovarian function. In general, after treatment for lymphoma, patients are advised to wait 1–2 years before attempting pregnancy. Whether this reduces risk is not clear, but appears sensible in the context of possible relapse.

Placental blood banking

It has been recognized for at least 30 years that hematopoietic transplantation was possible using fetal blood (50–150ml) obtained from the placental cord. This is possible due to the presence of mononuclear cells in the cord blood which can restore hematopoiesis in the treatment of a number of hematological malignancies, platelet and sickling disorders. Although many of the ethical and consent issues surrounding this modality of therapy are not yet resolved, there is an increasing demand for the provision of such cord stem cells for the management of hematological and, in the future, non-hematological conditions (Table 3.12).

Table 3.12 – Considerations in cord stem cell collection

Ethics/consent
Viral safety
Genetic disorder exclusion
Microbial safety
Traceability
Storage safety and records
Dose suitable for pediatric cases
? ↓ Graft rejection
? ↓ GVHD

GVHD, Graft-versus host disease

The criteria for the selection of maternal donors for allogenic donation are similar to those employed by most blood banking organizations, but with additional information required regarding past obstetric history and the possibility of transmission of genetic defects. A number of practical issues, such as the safety and yield of cells obtained when the cord is clamped early, or when the collection is taken prior to delivery of the placenta, are yet to be resolved. In addition, the effect of Cesarean, rather than vaginal, delivery on the quality of cells also requires further study. Overall, the collection appears to have little impact on staff time, with often only an additional 10 minutes required for such collections.

The testing of such donations covers similar areas to that of blood donation, including statutory virological screening (including hepatitis A, B and C, and HIV, human T-cell leukemia/lymphoma virus (HTLV) and cytomegalovirus (CMV)) and microbiological culture. The problem of window period infections and the absence of the safety net that is presumed to come from those who have successfully donated before, may all have an impact on the implementation of such placental banking programs.

In addition, there is the requirement (as with hematopoietic stem cells derived from adults) to determine the viability (from progenitor cell culture) and stem cell component of each collection. It has been supposed that the human leukocyte antigens (HLA) match may be less stringent with cord stem cells, although further work on this, and the exclusion of maternal cells from the collection, is required.

At present, cord banking remains an expensive source of hematopoietic stem cells, which, like cells derived from adults, requires a substantial infrastructure to maintain safety and traceability. To date, a substantial number of pediatric transplants have been carried out using cord stem cells, although much work is required to allow these collections to form the basis of transplants for adults. Ultimately, the expense of the collection and storage procedures may be offset by the greater amount of transplant material available from this source and (if confirmed) the requirement for less stringent HLA matching and lesser likelihood of graft-versus host disease with such transplants.

CHAPTER 4

Bleeding disorders in pregnancy

Hemophilia A

The gene coding for Factor (F) VIII is found on the X chromosome at position q28, and heritable deficiency of FVIII occurs as an X-linked recessive disorder. The frequency of hemophilia A is between 1 in 10 000 and 1 in 20 000 of the population. Although it has a wide distribution amongst different ethnic groups, it is rare in Chinese populations. The disorder results from a variety of genetic mutations, although 40% of severely affected individuals have an inversion involving intron 22 of the gene. By contrast, the majority of mild disease results from point mutations.

Clearly, this is a disorder predominantly affecting males; females will usually be heterozygous and therefore can only be carriers. For a karyotypically normal woman to have a hemorrhagic problem with hemophilia A, she would have to be either homozygous for the mutation (with inheritance of affected X chromosomes from both an affected father and a carrier mother – an exceptionally rare occurrence), or demonstrate significant lyonization (see below), with resulting low FVIII levels. The latter is not unusual in carriers, but virtually all carriers in this situation have levels of FVIII above that which would result in spontaneous bleeding problems. Moreover (see Chapter 1), the vast majority of such reduced FVIIIc levels will normalize during pregnancy. Other mechanisms of clinical FVIII deficiency in a female include an acquired antibody to FVIII, a hemophilia carrier with Turner's syndrome (XO), and autosomal dominant hemophilia A (due to a somatic gene affecting FVIII synthesis).

Hemophilia A tends to follow a similar pattern in affected family members, reflecting the particular genetic mutation associated with hemophilia A in their family, although in 30% of cases there may be no known family history. Daughters of an affected male are obligate carriers of the disease. Most of these will be unaffected unless there is extreme lyonization. Lyonization is the random inactivation of the X chromosome that occurs in all cells. If, by chance, this inactivation affects more of the normal X chromosome in FVIII-producing cells, this will produce a mild hemophilia state in the affected female carriers. A carrier female has a 50:50 chance of passing hemophilia onto her son and a 50:50 chance of passing the carrier state onto her daughter.

Presentation and treatment of affected males

Hemophilia results in a lifelong tendency to bleeding. In a severely affected male, symptoms are often first noted when he begins to crawl or walk. It is unusual to see bleeding problems in the neonate, including bleeding from the umbilical stump.

Symptoms are directly related to the level of remaining FVIIIc activity. A level of <1IU/dl leads to severe spontaneous bleeding, 1–5IU/dl to moderate bleeding only after minor trauma and 6–40IU/dl leading to mild bleeding only after major trauma.

The first episode of joint bleeding (hemarthrosis) often leads to future bleeding into the same joint (a target joint), resulting in arthropathy and joint failure. Any joint may be affected, although the knee is the most common site, with ankles, elbows, hips, shoulders and wrists also affected. Recurrent intramuscular, subcutaneous and intraperitoneal hematomas may occur. There may also be bleeding from the gastrointestinal (GI) tract, and bleeding after major trauma and dental extraction is a common problem. In such circumstances delayed bleeding is also common.

The diagnosis may be suspected if there is a prolongation of the activated partial thromboplastin time (APTT), although a normal time does not exclude mild disease. The diagnosis can be confirmed by determining the FVIIIc level by an APTT- or chromogenic-based test (a chromogenic test determines the level of FVIIIc by its ability to generate FXa from FXc, with the amount of FXa released detected by a quantifiable color change in the reaction mix). In all cases of severe hemophilia the level of FVIII antigen (determined by enzyme-linked immunosorbent assay (ELISA)) will also be reduced. In milder cases, there may

Table 4.1 – Diagnosis of hemophilia

	Hemophilia A	Hemophilia B	Hemophilia C	von Willebrand's disease	Lupus inhibitor
PT	√	√	√	√	√/ ↑
APTT	↑/√	↑/√	↑/√	Mild ↑	↑/√
TCT	√	√	√	√	√
APTT 50:50 mix	APTT corrects	APTT corrects	APTT corrects	APTT corrects	Poor/ no correction
FVIIIc	↓	√	√	Mild ↓	–
FIXc	√	↓	√	√	–
FXIc	√	√	↓	√	–
vWF	√/ ↑	√	√	↓	–

APTT, Activated partial thromboplastin time; F, Factor; PT, Prothrombin time; TCT, Thrombin clotting time; vWF, von Willebrand's Factor.

be a disparity between antigen and activity (i.e. activity that is less than antigen level), indicating the presence of a functional genetic defect. In most severe cases the only likely alternative diagnosis is either hemophilia B (FIX deficiency) or C (FXI deficiency). Thus, the initial diagnostic work-up should include an assay of FVIIIc, FIXc and FXIc. In milder cases, von Willebrand's disease (vWD) may also have to be excluded (Table 4.1). When the disease presents with the incidental finding of a prolonged APTT, a specific factor inhibitor (see below) or a lupus inhibitor (lupus anticoagulant) may have to be excluded.

General principles of treatment

In general, hemophilia treatments should be initiated under the supervision of a physician experienced in the management of hemophilia. In the UK there is a system of regional hemophilia centers, and patients with hemophilia will usually attend these centers or associated hospitals. In all cases, if a patient presents for care, the center responsible for the patient's hemophilia care should be contacted to determine the treatment product usually used and to ascertain if the patient is known to have a FVIII inhibitor, as this may influence the dose required to achieve the desired increment.

Factor replacement

Replacement with factor products in hemophilia A should be achieved with recombinant or high purity FVIII preparations where possible, with a dosage based upon the plasma concentration of FVIII required and upon the body weight or plasma volume. To calculate the required dose by weight the following formula can be used: (body weight [kg] × desired rise in FVIII [IU/100ml])/2. The amount of FVIII administered is expressed in IU: 1IU of FVIIIc equals the quantity of FVIIIc in 1ml of normal human plasma. Empirically, 1IU of FVIII/kg of body weight increases the plasma FVIIIc level by 1.5–2.0IU/100ml. After each dose a peak level should be checked and further doses given, if required, to maintain the target level (Table 4.2). When there has been bleeding, dose calculation by plasma volume may be more appropriate. When required, the plasma volume can be derived from the patient's hematocrit and their blood volume (which can be estimated as 7% of the body weight). For most clotting factors, the decline of therapeutic levels occurs in two phases: a rapid loss followed by a slower decline. For FVIII infusions, around 80% of the dose can be recovered initially in the plasma, leading to an initial and subsequent half-life of infused FVIII of 6 and 12 hours, respectively. This leads to a requirement to dose every 8–12 hours.

Because of repeated exposure to allogenic FVIII, the development of acquired inhibitors to FVIII is not uncommon in hemophilia A. In such circumstances, cross-reactivity of the antibody with porcine FVIII should be determined. Where there is little or no cross-reaction, porcine FVIII products can be used. This

Table 4.2 – Factor (F) VIII dosing in hemophilia A (HA) and hemophilia B (HB)

Bleeding	Target FVIIIc (IU/dl) or FIXc (U/dl)	Dosage frequency	Dose duration
Minor surgery	30–60	1/day	≥ 24 hours
Major surgery	80–100	1–3/day	Pre- and post-operative until adequate wound heal, then 30–60 IU/dl for <7 days
Early hemarthrosis Early muscle bleed Oral mucosa bleed	20–40	1–2/day HA 1/day HB	≥ 24 hours until resolution
Large hematoma Severe hemarthrosis	30–60	1–2/day HA 1/day HB	3–4 days until resolution
Life threatening (e.g. head injury)	60–100	1–3/day	Bleeding stopped

product is itself, however, associated with the possibility of antibody formation and mild thrombocytopenia is also not uncommon during dosing.

Desmopressin analog, DDAVP

In mild hemophilia A, all cases should have an assessment of the effect of DDAVP. DDAVP, when infused intravenously over 20 minutes at a dose of 0.3µg/kg diluted in 50–100ml of saline, will increase plasma FVIIIc and von Willebrand Factor (vWF) by 2–5 times above the basal level in around 30–60 minutes.

Patients with a basal level of FVIIIc or vWF of 10–20IU/dl are most likely to have a useful therapeutic response to DDAVP. In such subjects, the infusion can be repeated 12–24 hourly as required, although there is often a marked diminution of response after around 3 days (presumably due to depletion of vWF or FVIIIc stores, i.e. tachyphylaxis). DDAVP is therefore suitable for minor bleeds or minor surgical procedures where prolonged bleeding (>3 days) is unlikely. The drug is also available for subcutaneous or intranasal use. The intranasal spray gives a dose of 150µg/ml and should be given as a single dose of 300µg. Side effects of intravenous DDAVP include hypotension, flushing (which is common and appears to be due to prostacyclin release), tachycardia, headache, and, rarely, volume overload and hyponatremia. On repeated use it may be worth checking urea and electrolytes, and the product should be used with caution in those at risk of cardiac overload, fluid retention or hypertension.

Whether the increase in vWF and FVIII induced by DDAVP carries a thrombotic risk is not proven, but it should be used with caution in individuals with atherosclerosis or a high risk of thrombosis. When using DDAVP a further sample should be obtained 3–6 hours after dosing to determine that an adequate duration of response has occurred. Theoretically, DDAVP used at delivery could carry an increased risk of fetal hyponatremia. If this is a concern, then restricting use until after clamping the placental cord will avoid such a problem.

Antifibrinolytic agents

For minor surgery, antifibrinolytic agents (such as tranexamic acid) can be a useful adjunct to other therapy, and may be particularly useful in dental surgery. Tranexamic acid binds to plasminogen, inhibiting the binding of plasminogen to fibrin. This leads to a reduction in fibrinolysis, and has a plasma half-life of around 2 hours. It should be given in advance of any procedure and can be given as an oral dose, or as a mouthwash for dental procedures.

Renal tract bleeding and/or renal failure are contraindications to such therapies, as thrombosis in the renal tract may further impair renal function. Tranexamic acid should also be used with caution in pregnancy, as fibrinolysis is already shut down by the physiological increase in plasminogen activator inhibitor (PAI)-1 and PAI-2 (see Chapter 1).

Carrier detection in pregnancy

In an ideal world, potential carriers would be identified before pregnancy and counseling offered. In general, the phenotype of hemophilia A remains constant in families, and carriage of a mild defect should result in a mildly affected son. A mother is an obligate carrier of hemophilia if she has an affected father. She is also considered a carrier if she has had two affected sons, or if she has a family history and one affected son. It is also likely if she has no family history but has had an affected son.

A reduced level of FVIIIc is consistent with carriage of hemophilia, although, especially if an individual is pregnant or taking hormone therapy, a normal level does not exclude it. In suspected cases with a normal FVIIIc, it has been shown that the ratio of plasma FVIIIc:vWF levels may help distinguish between carriers and non-carriers, but this usually requires repeated examinations for confirmation; and it is unlikely to give useful information in pregnant subjects due to the marked physiological changes in both factors.

There are two types of genetic diagnosis that can be achieved: direct and indirect evidence of a mutation. In severe hemophiliacs, direct detection of the intron 22 inversion, or of another common inversion in part of the intron 22 sequence that is found telomeric to the gene, should be carried out. In mildly affected individuals, linkage analysis of polymorphisms can be carried out. This is the indirect method, which requires information from several family members, one of whom is required to carry the disease, and relies upon normally occurring variations in the genetic nucleotide sequence that can be used to track the mutant gene. Tracking is achieved by identifying the effect of these variations on enzyme-restriction sites in the gene in different family members. The polymorphisms often used are those involving the CA-repeat in intron 13, or other intragenic polymorphisms such as Bcl1, HindIII, Xba1, Bg1, Msp1 and Taq1. Which one is informative depends upon its frequency in the ethnic population under study.

Alternatively, direct sequencing of the FVIIIc promoter, exons and splice junctions will give diagnostic information in the majority of subjects.

Prenatal and pre-implantation diagnosis

In those many cases which are sporadic, elimination of hemophilia will not be possible by prenatal diagnosis. However, prenatal diagnosis can be achieved by a number of techniques. Of these, chorionic villus sampling (CVS) is commonly used.

CVS can be performed between 11 and 13 weeks gestation and carries around a 1% risk of fetal loss. Also, as it is carried out prior to the possibility of fetal sexing by ultrasound, CVS may result in unnecessary risk to a female fetus. In addition, CVS carried out earlier than 11 weeks can be associated with the development of fetal limb abnormality. CVS is used to determine the fetal sex in the first instance, with a result possible within 24 hours of sampling. Where appropriate, a known mutation can then be detected by sequencing within 7–10 days.

When a number of other family members are available (including an affected individual), restriction length fragment polymorphism can lead to a diagnosis of carriage within a few days, as there is no need to culture cells before analysis. The sample can be obtained by a transvaginal or transabdominal route. Genetic diagnosis by CVS is not, however, infallible, as there is always the possibility of contamination of the sample with maternal tissue and the possibility of mosaicism.

In the second trimester, it is usual to offer fetal sexing by ultrasound at around 18 weeks gestation. Amniocentesis can also be used to acquire fetal genetic material. Cordocentesis to determine fetal levels of FVIIIc or FIXc can be used between 18 and 20 weeks, but is often seen as a last resort, as it may lead to the stress of a later termination. Cordocentesis also carries a 1–3% risk of fetal loss. With such investigations, the possibility of immunization of RhD-negative women should always be considered and anti-D prophylaxis offered. Interestingly, the uptake of prenatal diagnosis and termination of affected pregnancies is relatively low (35 and 50%, respectively), since many carriers of hemophilia, who have family experience of the disorder, do not consider it to be sufficiently disabling to justify termination.

In the future the diagnosis may be achieved by isolation of fetal cells from the maternal circulation. At present this has been achieved by the sexing of fetal lymphocytes in the maternal circulation. As such lymphocytes are often long lasting this technique may only be applicable to primigravida. Other techniques, such as detection and genetic analysis of fetal normoblasts or trophoblast in the maternal circulation, are still in development.

The technology of assisted conception now offers the opportunity for pre-implantation genetic diagnosis, so avoiding the need for termination. Following ovulation induction and transvaginal ultrasound-guided oocyte retrieval, in vitro fertilization is performed, and single-cell biopsy at the 4–8 cell stage allows determination of the embryonic sex (usually by fluorescent in situ hybridization). This allows the potentially affected developing male embryos from a carrier mother, or the potential carrier female embryos of an affected male father, to be discarded and only unaffected embryos replaced, so avoiding the birth of an affected male or carrier female. The success rate for pregnancies following this procedure is consistent with other assisted reproduction techniques, and currently is of the order of 25–30%. There appears to be no developmental problem with the embryo when biopsied at this stage. This technique is now available in a limited number of centers in Europe and North America. In the future, more precise genetic testing on single cells may become more readily available, which will allow determination of whether the embryo carries the particular hemophilia gene for that family.

Antepartum carrier management

The levels of vWF and FVIIIc increase with gestation (see Chapter 1). On account of this, replacement products are rarely required in hemophilia A carriers antepartum. However, when early complications such as miscarriage or ectopic pregnancy occurs, or a procedure such as amniocentesis or CVS is required in a carrier, problems are occasionally seen. This is due to the lack of time for the physiological increase in FVIIIc to have occurred. If there is the potential for use of blood products (including recombinant products) during the pregnancy, then the woman should have her immunity to hepatitis A (HAV) and B (HBV) checked. If necessary, she should be immunized against HBV (and probably HAV), subcutaneously. It is safe to immunize her against HBV during the pregnancy. As the HAV vaccine is inactivated, it is also probably safe to use in pregnancy, but an assessment of the risk:benefit ratio depends upon the risk of contamination of HAV by locally available blood and blood products. FVIIIc levels should be checked in all carriers at the first antenatal visit and again in the third trimester. A level of 40IU/dl is usually sufficient to avoid hemorrhagic problems in early pregnancy and for a vaginal delivery. A level of ≥50IU/dl is required for diagnostic procedures, such as amniocentesis, Cesarean section or epidural anesthesia. Despite a lack of significant oxytocic effects, DDAVP is often avoided antepartum in mothers who have not demonstrated an adequate increase in FVIIIc levels. This is due to its association, in repeated doses, with maternal hyponatremia. However, it is usually preferable to blood products and it is unusual for repeated doses to be required. Moreover, it should be remembered that repeated doses are associated with tachyphylaxis and are less likely to give a useful clinical response. In the small number of carrier cases, where factor treatment is required, this should be with recombinant factors if at all possible.

Management of delivery and puerperium

On admission to the labor suite, a full blood count, coagulation screen, appropriate factor level assessment (unless these have previously been normal) and a cross-match sample for 'group-and-save' should be taken. Intramuscular analgesia should be avoided if the mother has a FVIII level <40IU/dl, but such therapy can be given intravenously.

The management of delivery must consider the possibility of fetal hemophilia. Even if the fetus is a female, it is important to remember that she may still be at risk of bleeding because of the combination of lyonization and the immaturity of the fetal liver with reduced coagulation factor production. In an attempt to 'boost' production of vitamin K-dependent coagulation factors from the fetal liver, many authorities prescribe vitamin K supplements (20mg/day) to the mother from 36 weeks gestation (or earlier if premature delivery is considered a possibility). Generally, vaginal delivery is preferred for known hemophilia carriers, with few obstetricians recommending Cesarean section purely on the basis of suspected (or known) fetal hemophilia. However, the main concern is of fetal intracerebral bleeding in the course of delivery. Where the fetus may be a carrier female or an affected male, it is prudent to avoid procedures that would place the fetus at increased risk of bleeding. 'Difficult' forceps deliveries, rotational forceps, ventouse extraction, scalp electrodes or fetal scalp blood sampling should be avoided. A straightforward mid- or low-cavity forceps delivery is usually considered to carry a reasonable risk. If, however, there is a delay in labor and an easy vaginal delivery seems less likely, the mother should be delivered by Cesarean section.

As pregnancy FVIIIc levels fall quickly to pre-pregnancy levels post-partum hemorrhage is possible, and FVIII levels should be maintained >40IU/dl for at least 3–4 days after vaginal delivery and for 4–5 days following Cesarean section. However, it is unusual for carriers to require postpartum management with DDAVP or FVIII concentrates. DDAVP can be used, if required, in breastfeeding mothers, as it does not cross the breast.

For the newborn, a cord determination of FVIIIc levels, on blood aspirated by clean venepuncture form the umbilical vein, should be obtained in all suspected or known cases if possible. Vaccines should be given by the subcutaneous route, and intramuscular injections and heel stabs (such as for the Guthrie test) avoided until the level of clotting factors is known. In such cases, vitamin K prophylaxis is routinely given by the oral rather than intramuscular route. Follow-up for determination and, if required, treatment must be organized with the appropriate pediatric hemophilia center.

Difficulties arise when a sporadic case of hemophilia unexpectedly presents with an intracerebral hemorrhage following vaginal delivery. In this context it is important to remember that approximately one third of cases of hemophilia are due to new mutations. In sporadic cases, hemophilia in the child may not be immediately considered and the mild prolongation of the APTT (which occurs in moderately affected individuals) may be interpreted as being within normal limits for the newborn. In all suspected cases, specific assays for FVIII should be carried out. Early prophylaxis after birth is often carried out if there has been an instrumental delivery. In some areas, serial brain ultrasounds are used to screen for intracerebral hemorrhage; screening for congenital dislocation of the hip is carried out with caution, or postponed until the results of factor levels are known.

Hemophilia B

Hemophilia B is another X-linked bleeding disorder, which, although considerably less common than hemophilia A, is more often associated with a family history. Hemophilia B may result from mutations that lead to a reduction in FIX function, accompanied by either detectable, or reduced, FIX antigen levels. The wide variety of mutations of the FIX gene includes those that alter carboxyl group formation (carboxyl groups on vitamin K-dependent factors lead to binding of the coagulation factor to activated phospholipid at the site of coagulation, accelerating the coagulation response) and those that alter the activation of FIXc by FXIa. In addition, a mutation in the FIX promoter region may lead to a marked reduction in antigen at birth, but increasing production occurs with increasing age (hemophilia B Leyden).

Severe FIX deficiency is considerably less common than severe hemophilia A, but presents with similar problems as hemophilia A subjects with comparable factor levels. The diagnosis of hemophilia B can be achieved by determination of FIXc in an APTT-based assay.

General principles of treatment

As with hemophilia A, treatment of hemophilia B should be supervised by a physician experienced in hemophilia management and in collaboration with the center responsible for the patient's long-term care.

When FIX is infused, only 50% is recovered initially, and the initial and subsequent half-lives are 3 and 24 hours, respectively. This means that FIX treatment requires a loading dose for immediate effect (even in minor bleeds), but subsequent doses can be given at 24-hour intervals. The treatment of choice is recombinant FIX, although this may require a higher dose than human-derived equivalents (see Table 4.2). Empirically, infusion of 1IU of human-derived FIX per kg of body weight increases the plasma FIXc level by 0.8% of normal activity. The required dose to be given can be calculated by: (body weight [kg] × the desired rise in FIXc [%]) × 1.2. If not available, other products, such as prothrombin concentrates (usually containing FIX, FX, FII +/-FVII), may have to be used. The dose is again calculated from the level of FIXc in such products. Aside from these factors, the principles of therapy and management in pregnancy are the same as for hemophilia A (see Table 4.2).

In subjects with complete absence of the FIX antigen, allergic reactions to factor products can be problematic. In such cases, therapy with recombinant FVIIa is a possible alternative. In the future it is hoped than gene therapy may have a role in the management of hemophilia B.

Pregnancy management

There is substantial genetic heterogeneity in cases of hemophilia B, with many mutations being peculiar to an individual family. Confirmation of female carriage requires knowledge of the mutation within the family to confirm the diagnosis. In general, to be certain that an identified mutation causes hemophilia, it is recommended that the clinician confirms that the mutation is already included in one of the international databases of hemophilia mutations. This is necessary, as a number of mis-sense mutations result in no observable change in the function of the FIX molecule. Furthermore, where there is a sporadic case, the mother may have a mosaic (a mixture of native and mutated DNA in the same germ cell) and carrier status cannot be confirmed by assessment of her somatic cells.

Female carriage is likely if there is a reduced level of FIX activity (which often results in a more clear-cut distinction from non-carriers than FVIII carriage in hemophilia A), but assessment of FIX antigen levels is more problematic, as there may be a considerable overlap with non-hemophilic subjects. Although FIX activity is higher in women on the combined oral contraceptive pill, it does not change substantially with increasing gestation, and those carriers with a low level tend not to 'nomalize' in pregnancy, in contrast to hemophilia A carriers.

All carriers should have an assessment of FIX levels at their first visit in pregnancy and in the third trimester. In more markedly affected carriers, hemostatic support is more likely to be required during pregnancy than with equivalent hemophilia A carriers. Such support should be with recombinant factor products, as DDAVP is usually ineffective in FIX deficiency. As with FVIII carriers, a FIX level of at least 40 U/dl is required for a vaginal delivery, and a level of at least 50 U/dl for Cesarean section or epidural. Levels should be maintained for the first 4–5 days after delivery.

The methods of prenatal diagnosis of FIX deficiency, and the management of the delivery and the postpartum phase, follow the same principles and techniques as those used for cases of FVIII deficiency. To facilitate restriction fragment length polymorphism (RFLP) detection, *Taq*1, *Xmn*1, *Dde*1, *Hha*1, *Mnl*1 and *Mse*1 are informative in around 90% of cases in Caucasians.

Hemophilia C

Hemophilia C is characterized by a reduction in coagulation FXIc. Unlike hemophilia A and B, it is inherited as an autosomal recessive trait. In homozygotes, the FXIc level may be <20 U/dl: in heterozygous subjects the levels range between 20 and 70 U/dl. The disorder has a prevalence in the general population of around one in one million, but occurs at a higher frequency in the Ashkenazi and Iraqi Jew populations, where up to 0.3% of subjects are homozygous for the deficiency and there is a gene prevalence of up to 11%.

The gene coding for FXI is found on chromosome 4, with at least 28 known mutations. These can result in an alteration of gene splicing (Type I mutations), the production of a stop codon (which leads to FXIc of <1U/dl), or a minor amino acid substitution (Type III mutations). Of these, mutations associated with the production of a stop codon (so-called Type II mutations) are most often associated with bleeding. In the Ashkenazi Jew population, two mutations are responsible for most cases, and compound Type II/Type III heterozygotes are the commonest cause of moderate to severe disease. In other populations there is a greater variation in the mutations involved.

Unlike hemophilia A and B, bleeding is more difficult to predict in subjects with hemophilia C. Generally, hemarthrosis is uncommon and spontaneous bleeding is rare. Furthermore, bleeding does not correlate well with residual FXI activity and around 50% of heterozygous subjects may have a bleeding tendency. By contrast, subjects with severe deficiency may not have a severe bleeding tendency. In many affected individuals bleeding only occurs following surgery or trauma. The possibility of delayed hemorrhage should be considered, especially in oral, ear, nose and throat (ENT), gynecological and urological surgery, where there is high local fibrinolytic activity.

FXI deficiency may prolong the APTT, although this is only likely to detect homozygous subjects. In all suspected cases, a FXIc assay should be performed.

Management in pregnancy

As with other heritable bleeding disorders, pregnant subjects should be managed in a center with expertise in the assessment and treatment of hemophilia.

There are a variety of studies that show no change in FXIc levels with gestation in normal individuals, although many show a gradual reduction. As there is no good correlation between FXIc levels and bleeding in hemophilia C, close monitoring of FXIc levels in pregnancy in hemophilia C subjects is of doubtful value in any case.

Postpartum hemorrhage occurs in 20% of homozygotes, but excessive bleeding may also occur in heterozygotes. In general, the majority of subjects with a non-pregnant FXIc level of <15U/dl are likely to suffer excessive bleeding after trauma or surgery, and any subject who has a history of excessive blood loss will require hemostatic support for delivery. Even if specific hemostatic support is thought not to be required, products should be available.

When therapy is needed, daily use of a FXI concentrate is probably justified, with the aim of achieving a target FXIc level of no >70IU/dl (maximum dose of 30IU/kg). This level should be achieved during labor and maintained for 3–4 days after vaginal delivery and 4–5 days after Cesarean section.

The target level of FXIc should not exceed 100U/dl, as this has been associated with thrombosis, although it is not known whether there is an excessive risk of thrombosis whilst using FXI concentrates in late pregnancy and the puerperium. Although many manufacturers have added heparin to FXI concentrates, since the early reports of thrombosis, it is not yet clear that this has reduced the thrombotic potential of these products. In subjects with a history of thrombosis or atherosclerosis, FXI concentrate should probably be avoided. If hemostatic support is required, then fresh frozen plasma (FFP) should be used (FFP should be virally inactivated if at all possible).

If there has been no history of bleeding, tranexamic acid could be used to cover delivery in the first instance. However, as noted earlier, fibrinolysis is already impaired in pregnancy and tranexamic acid should be used with caution in view of the potential for thrombosis. There should be early recourse to FXI concentrate, if available, when treatment is needed. While FFP is an alternative, the use of FFP in such circumstances is complicated by the relatively large volume required and the variable half-life of the coagulation factors within it. Similarly, if, in an emergency, FXI products are not available, then FFP should be used if hemostatic support is required. The role of recombinant FVIIa is not yet certain, although it has been used effectively in subjects with FXI inhibitors, and it may be preferable to the use of human blood products in pregnancy.

If regional anesthesia is required, correction of the APTT has been advocated, although this remains controversial. As with any other hemophilia, the possibility of fetal carriage should be considered when planning fetal monitoring, forceps and ventouse extraction at delivery.

Acquired hemophilia

Acquired hemophilia results from the development of an autoantibody, most often against FVIII. Although classically associated with repeated treatment with allogenic factor products in subjects with hemophilia, it can also occur in normal healthy individuals, in subjects with autoimmune disorders (such as systemic lupus erythematosis (SLE) and rheumatoid arthritis (RA)), in those with lymphoproliferative and solid tumors, as well as in association with pregnancy. In non-hemophilia subjects it is a rare and sporadic disorder, and the incidence has been estimated at between 0.2 and 1 per million person-years. Of these, around 10% occur in relation to pregnancy.

Presentation in pregnancy

Pregnancy-related cases are often diagnosed within 3 months of delivery, although presentation up to 1 year after delivery has been reported. Presentation varies from bleeding after surgical procedures to spontaneous bruising, widespread hematomas and GI bleeding. If untreated, acquired hemophilia carries a substantial morbidity and mortality. Unlike inherited hemophilia, the bleeding tendency does not equate well with the level of inhibitor, and although GI bleeding is more common, joint hemarthrosis rarely occurs. In cases associated with pregnancy, the presentation may often be with a postpartum hemorrhage, although maternal fatality has been reported in association with retroperitoneal and respiratory tract bleeding.

The diagnosis is suspected if there is unexpected bleeding and evidence of a prolonged APTT which does not correct with the addition of normal plasma (most easily achieved by testing a 1:1 mixture of the patient and normal plasma). A prolonged APTT that corrects with normal plasma, indicates a clotting factor deficiency. If the APTT fails to correct, presence of either a coagulation factor inhibitor (antibody) or a lupus inhibitor (lupus anticoagulant) is indicated. The degree of inhibitor level is assessed by the Bethesda assay. Acquired inhibitors can be directed at any clotting factor, although FVIII inhibitors are most often recognized.

Treatment in pregnancy

The management of these patients requires consideration of both the level of inhibitor and the clinical problem. In those with a high level of inhibitor (Bethesda >10U), the therapeutic options include porcine FVIII, recombinant FVIIa (rFVIIa), or activated clotting factor concentrates (e.g. FEIBA®) (Table 4.3). The potential value of porcine FVIII can be assessed by laboratory determination of cross-reactivity of the inhibitor with porcine FVIII. With low-level inhibitors, spontaneous resolution without immunosuppression often occurs. In some cases there may be no response to high-dose FVIII, even when a low titer of inhibitor is present: indeed, even high-level inhibitors can sometimes respond to normal doses of FVIII.

The 2-year mortality has been estimated at 3%, with complete resolution of the antibody in almost all survivors by this time. Indeed, commonly, resolution occurs 6 weeks to 6 months after presentation. The use of immunosuppression may shorten the duration of the disease, but it is not yet clear whether it influences mortality. From the little information that is available, it appears that there is unlikely to be a recurrence in a future pregnancy. If a recurrence does occur, antepartum bleeding appears to be uncommon. In the vast majority of such cases the fetus is not affected, although sporadic case reports of low FVIII levels in the infant of an affected mother and of intracranial hemorrhage have been reported.

von Willebrand's disease (vWD)

vWF is required to bind platelets to the subendothelium upon vessel injury. The non-covalent binding of vWF to FVIII in the plasma also protects FVIII from degradation. Indeed, without vWF, the half-life of FVIII is reduced to a few

Table 4.3 – Management of acquired hemophilia

Bethesda <5U	High-dose human FVIII High-dose recombinant FVIII	Spontaneous resolution likely	Expensive
Bethesda >10U	Porcine FVIII	Good response likely, little cross-reaction with most inhibitors	Risk of allergy/ anaphylaxis/ thrombocytopenia
	Recombinant VIIa	Good response likely	Expensive Risk of thrombosis
	Activated clotting factor concentrate	Response can be measured clinically only	Risk of thrombosis Risk of disseminated intravascular coagulation (DIC)
	Additional therapy	Corticosteroids Cyclophosphamide Human normal intravenous immunoglobulin (IVIgG) Azathioprine Plasma exchange	

hours, leaving FVIIIc levels of between 1 and 10IU/dl. vWD results in a reduction of vWF and is the most common heritable bleeding disorder, with a frequency that has been estimated at around 1% of many populations. Many mild cases remain undiagnosed, as subjects are often asymptomatic.

The gene coding for vWF is found on chromosome 12, and the vWF molecule is produced both in the megakaryocyte (the precursor of platelets) and in the endothelium. Upon manufacture, it is stored in the Weibel-Palade bodies of the endothelium and in the α granules of platelets. Upon release into the circulation, vWF is cleaved by a proteinase of the A disintegrin and metalloprotease with thrombospondin domain (ADAMTS) family to achieve the correct balance of vWF multimers (see Chapter 8).

A brief description of the various types of vWD is shown in Table 4.4. The variants range from a mild/partial deficiency to a severe deficiency; between these two extremes are other variants. Some reduce the interaction of vWF with platelets (associated with either reduced or normal levels of high-molecular-weight vWF multimers). One produces a variant vWF that has an increased affinity for platelets. This, somewhat paradoxically, results in bleeding associated with thrombocytopenia and increased clearance of high-molecular-weight vWF multimers. There is also a vWD variant that has a reduced interaction with FVIII: in this variant the reduction in the half-life of FVIII contributes to the bleeding phenotype.

Table 4.4 – Classification of von Willebrand's disease (vWD)

	Defect	Inheritance	Bleeding time	Plasma vWF	Plasma FVIIIc	RiCoF	Multimer analysis
Type 1	Mild deficiency	Aut dom	↑ /√	↓ /√	√/↓	√/↓	√
Type 2	↓ platelet-dependent vWF function (Type IIa)	Aut dom	↑	↓ /√	√/↓	↓	↓ High molecular weight
	↑ vWF affinity to platelet glycoprotein 1b → High-molecular-weight multimers (Type IIb)	Aut dom	↑	√/↓ (↑ Platelet affinity)	√/↓	√/↓	↓ High molecular weight
	↓ Platelet-dependent function	Aut dom	↑	↓ /√	√/↓	√/↓	√
	↓ vWF affinity to FVIII	Aut rec	↑	↓ /√	√/↓	√/↓	√
Type 3	Severe deficiency of vWF	Aut rec	↑	↓	↓	↓	Variable

Aut dom, Autosomal dominant; Aut rec, Autosomal recessive; F, Factor; RiCoF, Ristocetin cofactor; vWF, von Willebrand Factor.

Clinically, a reduction in vWF results in a defect of primary hemostasis. In severe vWD, the accompanying reduction in circulating FVIII also results in a mild–moderate hemophilia A phenotype. The problems of milder vWD can be summarized as bleeding from surfaces. This includes mennorrhagia, bruising, epistaxis, postpartum hemorrhage and bleeding after dental extraction. In such individuals the diagnosis may not be made until the patient is an adult. In more severe defects, the significant contribution from the deficiency of FVIII results in hematoma and hemarthrosis formation. In such severely affected females, bleeding may come to attention in childhood, with life-threatening epistaxis, and bruising and menstrual bleeding is often extremely problematic at the menarche.

Screening for defects in primary hemostasis often employs the 'bleeding time' in the first instance. This is the time taken for hemostasis (more properly, the time when there is no further visible change in bleeding from the wound) after a cut (ideally a pair of cuts, made in a uniform direction) has been made (by a standard blade, usually a springloaded device that cuts at uniform length and depth such as the Simplate II) on the forearm, where a blood pressure cuff is maintained at 40mmHg. The bleeding time is difficult to standardize and reference ranges are not known for many clinical circumstances. In normal non-pregnant subjects the bleeding time is <9 minutes, but it may not be prolonged in all subjects with vWD.

In all suspected cases, an assessment of the APTT, vWF antigen, vWF activity and FVIIIc should be carried out. As FVIIIc and vWF increase in inflammation and in response to estrogen, the diagnosis of mild vWD can be problematic. In such cases, multiple evaluations are often required to confirm the diagnosis. vWF antigen is usually determined by ELISA and function is most often assessed by the ristocetin cofactor (RiCoF) activity of the patient's vWF. Ristocetin activates the patient's vWF, which then binds to test platelets (not the patient's) via platelet receptor Glycoprotein 1b (GPIb). By contrast, ristocetin can also be used to test the response of patient platelets to ristocetin. This test is used to diagnose platelet GPIb deficiency (Bernard Soulier syndrome) and to detect the increased reactivity of patient platelets to vWF, which is seen in Type IIb vWD (see Table 4.4), and pseudo-vWD (due to the high affinity of platelet GP1b for vWF). Other tests of vWF function (such as FVIII binding) are limited to more specialized laboratories. In all cases of reduced vWF, multimer analysis (by gel electrophoresis) is required to allow subclassification of the disease.

General principles of treatment

Most Type 1 vWD, the commonest form of vWD, will respond to an infusion of the vasopressin analogue DDAVP (see page 69). By contrast, Type 3 disease will require infusion of a product containing vWF. Although such products also contain FVIII they result in a longer survival of FVIII than happens in equivalent hemophilia A patients, due to the stabilization of endogenous FVIII by the infused vWF. In Type 2a vWD, DDAVP may occasionally be useful, although vWF concentrates are often required. In Type 2b vWD there is often a mild thrombocytopenia, which often worsens in pregnancy and may fall in response to DDAVP. In such cases DDAVP should probably be avoided. In subjects who do not respond to DDAVP, treatment with a plasma-derived factor concentrate that contains both FVIII and vWF is required (an 'intermediate purity' FVIII concentrate). A rough guide to dosing is shown in Table 4.5. The adequacy of the dose can be assessed by monitoring either FVIIIc or vWF RiCoF levels. In some Type 2 vWD, RiCoF assessment is more useful, as the baseline FVIIIc is within reference limits. There is no practical role for monitoring the bleeding time, as it reflects platelet vWF rather than vWF in the plasma.

As noted above, tranexamic acid may be a useful adjunct to other therapy, and in particular has a role in dental procedures. Although cryoprecipitate contains up to 10 times more FVIII and vWF than FFP, unlike concentrates it undergoes no virucidal procedures, and the exact amounts of factor contained in each dose is unknown. Correspondingly, it should only be used in an emergency when a suitable intermediate FVIII concentrate cannot be obtained.

Where methylene blue (MB)-treated cryoprecipitate is available, this should be used in preference to an untreated version. MB is a cross-linking agent that destroys some of the known blood-borne viruses. In most recently developed products, >95% of the added MB is removed during product manufacture. The potential for MB treatment to reduce the level of FVIII and vWF in the product should, however, be borne in mind when dosing this product. In cases of Type 3 vWD that do not respond to vWF concentrates, a combination of vWF concentrate and platelet component therapy may prove useful.

Antenatal management

All women with vWD should be managed in a unit with rapid access to specialized hemophilia care. If the fetus is at risk of Type 3 vWD, prenatal diagnosis may be

Table 4.5 – Intermediate Factor (F) VIII dosing in von Willebrand's disease (vWD)

Condition		Required FVIII/ RiCoF (IU/dl)	Dosage frequency	Dose duration
Surgery	Minor	>30	1/day	≥ 24 hours
	Major	>50	1/day	On op day and post-op until adequate wound healing
	Dental extraction	>30	One dose pre-procedure	≥ 12 hours
Bleeding		>30	1/day	Until resolution

RiCoF, Ristocetin cofactor.

required. This requires planning to determine the mutation or RFLP, which may be informative. Although vWF levels increase with gestation, it is important to assess vWF and FVIIIc levels between 34 and 36 weeks gestation in all women with vWD, to confirm that the levels have increased sufficiently to allow labor and delivery without the need for DDAVP or blood products. In subjects with mild–moderate vWD (Types 1 and 2), vWF levels usually increase from the 6th to 10th weeks of gestation, increasing 3–4-fold by the third trimester, making antenatal therapy (as with hemophilia A carriers) unnecessary in most cases. Indeed, it appears that significant antepartum hemorrhages and miscarriages are no more common in such subjects. However, as with hemophilia A, early pregnancy complications may require specific treatment to improve vWF levels.

As discussed above, DDAVP, if required, has no significant oxytocic effects, is not associated with teratogenicity in animal studies and has been used in early pregnancy to permit CVS or amniocentesis. In Type 3 vWD there is no rise in vWF with gestation or DDAVP, and factor therapy may be required to cover interventional procedures or spontaneous bleeding. As noted above (page 70), tranexamic acid is not absolutely contraindicated in pregnancy and is not associated with teratogenicity.

Management of delivery

A vWF or FVIII activity level of >40IU/dl or >50IU/dl, respectively, is considered safe for vaginal delivery or Cesarean section (or other procedures such as amniocentesis or evacuation of the uterus). After delivery, the levels of vWF rapidly return to pre-pregnancy levels and so, in general, vWD is associated with a higher risk of primary and secondary postpartum hemorrhage. However, in most Type 1 and 2 vWD, prophylactic therapy for vaginal delivery is not needed, although treatment may be required for episiotomy or perineal tears in Type 2 disease. In Type 1 vWD, epidural analgesia should not be undertaken lightly, but with due regard to the risks of spinal hematoma. In those who are known to respond to DDAVP, this can be used to cover Cesarean section. Although there maybe a theoretical risk, it is not clear whether DDAVP use at delivery carries any increased risk of fetal hyponatremia. If this is a concern, then restricting use until after clamping the placental cord will avoid such a problem. In Type 1 vWD there will be a fall in vWF after delivery, and discharge planning in women with symptomatic disease should take account of the possibility of secondary postpartum hemorrhage (PPH) at 4–5 days after delivery. In any case, vWF and FVIIIc levels should be monitored in all cases in the first days after delivery. After Cesarean section, DDAVP or factor products (if they have been used) should be continued for at least the first 2–3 days of the puerperium.

Type 3 vWD is, however, often associated with intrapartum and postpartum hemorrhage. FVIIIc levels at delivery have been used as a guide to the necessity for therapy, although the prediction of bleeding (as with any delivery) is problematic. As a guide, if the patient's FVIIIc level is <20IU/dl, therapy may be required. In such cases, therapy should be given to cover the episiotomy, and daily therapy after vaginal or Cesarian section delivery should be continued for the first week of the puerperium. Simlarly, epidural anesthesis is not recommended for Type 2 or 3 disease.

As with all bleeding disorders, where a fetus is at risk of inheriting vWD, delivery should be managed to minimize the risk of trauma to the fetus. In all suspected cases, the umbilical cord venous level of vWF should be assessed with a sample obtained by clean venepuncture: it should be noted that this is not reliable for the exclusion of Type 1 disease. For some forms of Type 2 disease an assessment of cord FVIIIc is also required to establish or exclude disease.

Hypo- and Dysfibrinogenemia

Fibrinogen is synthesized by hepatocytes coded by three genes on chromosome 4. Fibrinogen functions as the precursor of fibrin clot, interacts with activated platelets and acts as a plasma carrier for FXIII. Two types of congenital fibrinogen disorder are recognized: those where the fibrinogen antigen is produced but is poorly functioning (dysfibrinogenemia), and those where there is a reduction (hypofibrinogenemia) or absence (afibrinogenemia) of the fibrinogen antigen.

Afibrinogenemia

Although afibrinogenemia, usually an autosomal recessive trait, can be associated with life-threatening hemorrhage, bleeding is usually less than that observed in hemophilia A and B. Bleeding may occur, however, from the umbilical stump and bleeding into joints is not uncommon, but bleeding from the GI tract and the central nervous system (CNS) is infrequently seen.

In affected mothers, there may be an increase in the risk of first trimester miscarriage, placental abruption and postpartum hemorrhage. In such circumstances, maternal fibrinogen replacement is often required for the pregnancy to proceed to term.

As fibrinogen is the final component of hemostasis, congenital afibrinogenemia can be suspected from a failure to clot in the prothrombin time (PT), APTT and thrombin clotting time (TCT). This is accompanied by an absence of fibrinogen antigen and, in some cases, a prolonged bleeding time.

When treatment is required, this should be achieved by a virus-inactivated fibrinogen concentrate where it is available. Where it is not, cryoprecipitate may have to be used (with the caveats noted above). Prophylaxis is indicated in pregnancy and fibrinogen levels should be restored to at least 1g/l. In afibrinogenemia, exposure to allogenic fibrinogen may result in allergy or anaphylaxis, and restoration of fibrinogen levels has also been associated with the development of thrombosis.

Hypo- and dysfibrinogenemia

Patients with hypofibrinogenemia and a fibrinogen level >0.5g/l are usually symptom free. As noted above, patients with a disparity between fibrinogen antigen and activity are described as dysfibrinogenemia. Such disparity may affect any aspect of fibrinogen function and, as a result, around 40% present with bleeding, around 40% are asymptomatic, and the remainder present with thrombosis or a combination of bleeding and thrombosis.

Dysfibrinogenemia may result in a prolongation of the TCT (and occasionally the PT), or, occasionally, shortening of the TCT. In all cases, the diagnosis requires the demonstration of a disparity between the fibrinogen activity and fibrinogen antigen levels. In many centers, a persistent ratio of >1.7 antigen:activity is considered to be in keeping with the diagnosis.

Congenital dysfibrinogenemia is most often inherited as an autosomal dominant trait, and should be distinguished from acquired dysfibrinogenemia associated with liver disease, malignancy and, disseminated intravascular coagulation (DIC). The majority of congenital cases require no therapy, but cryoprecipitate and antifibrinolytic agents have been used to prevent bleeding. Cryoprecipitate has also been used as prophylaxis in subjects who have suffered previous recurrent miscarriages, although evidence for this use is lacking. Because of the association of dysfibrinogenemia and thrombosis, many clinicians have a concern about using fibrinogen concentrate. However, in view of the limitations and risks of repeated cryoprecipitate exposure noted above, and the likelihood that more modern fibrinogen concentrates carry a lower thrombotic risk than older products, this is probably not justified, particularly if the patient has a history of hemorrhage rather than thrombosis.

Factor (F) XIII deficiency

As detailed in Chapter 1, FXIII is required for the stabilization of the fibrin clot. FXIII deficiency can occur as a very rare autosomally inherited disorder, which has a prevalence of around one in one million of Caucasian populations, but there is likely to be a higher prevalence where there is a large Asian population, or where there is a high incidence of consanguinity. As with other factor deficiencies, there is a relationship between the residual level of factor and bleeding risk. Allowing for differences in assay techniques, a level of <1IU/dl is associated with severe spontaneous bleeding and a level of 1–4IU/dl with a risk of moderately severe bleeding: levels >5IU/dl are most often asymptomatic, but bleeding episodes can occur. Affected individuals often present with bleeding from the umbilical stump in the first few days after delivery. In general, inheritance of the disorder produces a significant phenotype and, akin to more common hemophilias, is associated with bruising, muscle bleeding and hemarthrosis. There is also a lifelong increased risk of intracerebral hemorrhage, as well as bleeding after delivery, trauma and operative procedures. FXIII deficiency can also result in a delay in wound healing and has been associated with a high risk of recurrent miscarriage.

Diagnosis

In suspected cases, the PT, APTT and bleeding time will be normal. If suspected, a test to detect an abnormal solubility of fibrin can be used as a screening test for the disorder. This is carried out by clotting an anticoagulated patient sample with thrombin and calcium. The clot is then exposed to a chemical such as urea or acetic acid. Of these, acetic acid may have a greater sensitivity to milder defects (FXIII <10IU/dl) than urea (FXIII <5IU/dl), and is probably the more useful screening test. Such tests should be confirmed by a specific assay of FXIIIc levels. There are a number of FXIIIc assays available, although there is a great variation in their performance between different laboratories; an FXIII antigen assessment by ELISA is also available in some areas. Despite these variations, such tests will be of use in monitoring the response to therapy.

General principles of treatment

As it is generally recognized that significant FXIII deficiency carries a not insubstantial risk of intracerebral hemorrhage, all patients with severe FXIII deficiency (<1IU/dl) should be offered prophylaxis with FXIII concentrate from diagnosis. It should also be actively considered in those with milder deficiencies. FXIII has a long half-life of 7–10 days and 4-weekly dosing, at 10IU/kg, should be sufficient to maintain levels of between 3 and 10IU/dl: this level should be sufficient to prevent spontaneous hemorrhage. An acute bleed should be treated by a virus-inactivated concentrate (with a dose of 10–20IU/kg to maintain levels within normal limits until the bleeding has resolved), although FFP and cryoprecipitate have also been used successfully to manage hemorrhage. As platelets also contain FXIII, platelet therapy may also be helpful in an extreme emergency, if an appropriate product is not available.

Management in pregnancy

It has been reported that up to 50% of pregnancies in those with severe FXIII deficiency will result in miscarriage without therapy. It is, therefore, usual practice for all severely affected women who conceive to receive monthly infusions to maintain a FXIII trough level at >3IU/dl from the diagnosis of pregnancy.

As affected neonates may present with persistent bleeding from the umbilical cord, and are at risk of intracerebral bleeding, close collaboration is required with neonatologists to rapidly diagnose and treat infants presenting with unexplained hemorrhage in the presence of a normal coagulation screen and platelet count. This is particularly relevant if there is known to be consanguinity in the parents.

Ehlers Danlos syndromes

Mutations in some of the many genes which control collagen synthesis and metabolism can result in the variety of clinical patterns that are grouped together as Ehlers Danlos syndromes. The diagnosis is based upon the combination of clinical findings and family history, and six major clinical patterns are recognized. Each results in a variable combination of joint hyperextensibility, skin extensibility and skin fragility: the latter is associated with spontaneous bruising and the characteristic wide, poorly healed, papery scars which can occur on pressure areas. In Ehlers Danlos syndromes the clotting screen is normal and, despite the bruising tendency, the bleeding time and platelet function testing are most often normal. There are also associated cardiac abnormalities, which most often result in mitral valve prolapse, although, uncommonly there may be aortic dilatation. In addition, there may be associated retinal and dental problems. Such patients may be at increased risk of bleeding associated with delivery. Although there are no specific proven treatments, prolonged bleeding times can be improved with DDAVP in some cases, and there are case reports of a useful effect if DDAVP is given in such subjects prophylactically in the management of labor. As with other inherited disorders, there is a need to provide appropriate counseling as part of pre-pregnancy planning.

CHAPTER 5

Antithrombotic therapy in pregnancy

In pregnancy, it is critical to consider the effects of any drug, not only on the mother but also on the developing baby, e.g. teratogenesis in the first trimester, developmental problems in the second and third trimesters, delivery problems, and also the potential for longer term effects on childhood growth and development. In this regard, particular concerns exist in relation to anticoagulants and antithrombotic therapies in pregnancy, and a sound understanding of the efficacy and safety of these agents is essential in order to provide the optimal management of thrombotic problems in pregnancy.

Coumarins

Of the coumarin group of drugs, warfarin is commonly employed in a large number of countries. Warfarin is an orally active 4-hydroxycoumarin, which inhibits the synthesis of the vitamin K-dependent clotting and anticoagulant factors (see Table 5.1). This includes the coagulation factors (F) II, VII, IX and X, and the natural endogenous anticoagulants protein C and protein S. War-

Table 5.1 – The effect of warfarin

↓ Clotting factor activity	↓ FII, FVII, FIX, FX ↓ PS, PC	
Prothrombotic in first 24 hours	If initiated alone in VTE No risk if used for AF	
Target INR ([PT/PT$_c$]^{ISI})	2–3 DVT/AF 3–4 ArtT/mechanical valve/recurrent VTE	
Fetal risks	<12 (6–9) weeks 12–36 weeks >36 weeks	Embryopathy IQ and developmental defects ICH/abruption

AF, Atrial fibrillation; ArtT, Arterial thrombisis; DVT, Deep vein thrombosis; F, Factor; ICH, Intracerebral hemorrhage; INR, International normalized ratio; IQ, Intelligence quotient; ISI, International sensitivity index; PC, Protein C; PS, Protein S; PT, Prothrombin time; PTc, Control PT; VTE, Venous thromboembolism.

farin reduces the carboxylation of these factors, which renders them unable to bind to catalytic phospholipid, which in turn is required for successful coagulation (see Chapter 1). Warfarin has a long half-life, but its effect reflects the half-life of the vitamin K factors. When warfarin therapy is commenced there is an initial reduction in the levels of both FVIIc and protein S that is evident within around 6 hours, reflecting the short half-life of these factors. Indeed, it is this rapid fall in FVIIc that makes the prothrombin time (PT) useful in predicting the outcome of acute liver injury. However, on account of the rapid fall in protein S, warfarin, when used alone, may induce a pro-coagulant imbalance in the first days of therapy. This may lead to microvascular thrombosis and skin necrosis. The risk, however, appears to apply only to those subjects who have suffered thrombosis (when there may be consumption of coagulation and anticoagulant factors, and perhaps an underlying thrombophilia), but does not extend to those receiving warfarin as prophylaxis for atrial fibrillation. For this reason, heparin therapy should overlap with warfarin in the treatment of thrombosis until the international normalized ratio (INR: see below) is >2. The other vitamin K-dependent coagulation factors have considerably longer half-lives.

Warfarin is highly bound to albumin and is itself metabolized in the liver. The dose of warfarin given depends upon its measured effect on the PT (see Chapter 1), which is often reported as an INR. The INR compares the patient's PT (in seconds) with that of a normal pool of plasma. These clotting times are examined simultaneously by clotting the anticoagulated plasma samples with tissue factor (TF) and calcium. A ratio of the patient:normal pool plasma clotting time is generated. To allow inter-laboratory and international comparisons, the TF used should have a known sensitivity (called the international sensitivity index or (ISI)). To generate the INR, the patient:control ratio is then logged to the power of the ISI, e.g. for a thromboplastin with an ISI of 1.1, the INR would be equal to the (patient PT:control PT)$^{1.1}$. This allows the comparison of PT generated in different laboratories using different TF. In general, the nearer the ISI is to one, the more precise and safe the INR assessment will be.

A number of factors can interact with warfarin, resulting in an enhanced or reduced effect (Table 5.2). As a general rule, an INR of 2–3 is the aim for treatment of deep vein thrombosis (DVT), or for the prophylaxis of atrial fibrillation (often with a target INR of 2.5), and an INR of 3–4 (often with a target of 3.5) is the aim for the management of arterial thrombosis, mechanical heart valves or a venous thrombosis that has occurred despite an INR of 2–3.

On account of the individual variability of warfarin dosage, long-term warfarin carries a not insubstantial risk of bleeding, which after 6 months of treatment for a first DVT can be equivalent to the risk of DVT recurrence. This is why anticoagulation for DVT is restricted to 3–6 months of therapy, as after this time, in most cases, the risk of anticoagulation outweighs the risk of recurrent thrombosis.

Table 5.2 – Factors increasing anticoagulation and bleeding with warfarin

Patient factors		↑ Age
		Liver dysfunction
		Alcohol
		Cardiac failure
		Renal failure
		Weight loss/acute illness
Drug interaction	NSAID	↓ Clotting factor synthesis
		↓ Albumin binding
	Antibiotics	↓ Vitamin K absorption
		↓ Warfarin metabolism
		(e.g. erythromycin)
	Cimetidine	↓ Warfarin metabolism
	Phenytoin	↓ Clotting factor synthesis, but also
		↑ Warfarin metabolism
	Sodium valporate	↓ Warfarin metabolism
	Laxatives	↓ Vitamin K absorption
Additional anticoagulation		Aspirin
		Heparins
		Thrombolysis

NSAID, Non-steroidal anti-inflammatory drug.

Warfarin in pregnancy

Warfarin crosses the placenta and inhibits coagulation factor production by the fetal liver. It is also teratogenic, but is not found, to any significant degree, in breast milk and is therefore safe to use in breastfeeding mothers. In the first trimester, exposure to warfarin may result in warfarin embryopathy. The fetus is vulnerable between 6 and 9 weeks gestation, and the incidence has been estimated at around 6% of pregnancies exposed to warfarin in the first trimester. The effect appears to be dose (not INR) dependent, with an increased risk evident with does >5mg/day. Warfarin embryopathy can be avoided when warfarin is substituted by heparin between 6 and 12 weeks gestation. There is also, however, an association between warfarin usage and miscarriage, and around 25% of women taking warfarin throughout pregnancy will miscarry. Similar figures are seen even when heparin is substituted in the first trimester. However, if warfarin is discontinued and heparin employed at/or prior to 6 weeks gestation, the miscarriage rate drops to 15%. This emphasizes the critical nature of switching to heparin before 6 weeks gestation to obtain the maximal benefit.

Warfarin embryopathy results in chondrodysplasia punctata (nasal and midface hypoplasia, frontal bossing, short proximal limbs, scoliosis, short phalanges and short stature). There is also a characteristic facial appearance with nasal hypoplasia. This is due to warfarin-induced premature calcification of the nasal cartilage, which results in failure of growth of the nose during childhood development. This defect is, however, amenable to corrective plastic surgery. In addition, when warfarin has been used between 12 and 36 weeks gestation, an association has been reported between its use and neurological and developmental problems in the infant. It is supposed that this is due to small intracerebral bleeds in the fetus, consequent upon excessive anticoagulation (due to the immature status of the fetal liver). Indeed, intracerebral bleeds have been reported in the fetus of women treated with warfarin in the second and third trimesters. Between 36 weeks gestation and delivery, there may be an increased risk of abruption and of intracerebral bleeding in the fetus (particularly during delivery), as well as a risk of severe maternal bleeding at delivery.

Thus, although warfarin may be preferred to heparin in the maternal interest for some conditions (such as mechanical heart valves or severe recurrent thrombosis), due to the better efficacy data for preventing maternal thrombosis, it carries significant risks for the fetus. In each case it is critical to establish the optimal anticoagulation regime, balancing the risks between the mother and the fetus, and taking into account the mother's view of these risks. Such decisions are clearly best made prior to pregnancy. All women on oral anticoagulants who could become pregnant must be aware of the risks of conceiving whilst on these drugs, and of the need to report to their hematologist and/or high-risk obstetrician immediately they become pregnant to ensure that optimal anticoagulation and pregnancy management can be provided. In particular, as noted above, a switch to heparin should be made before 6 weeks gestation if this is the therapeutic strategy that is to be employed.

Heparin

The heparins are glycosaminoglycans with a high affinity for the endogenous anticoagulant antithrombin (see Chapter 1), altering both its structure and anticoagu-

Table 5.3 – Low-molecular-weight heparin (LMWH)

No effect on APTT	Even in overdose
Reversal may need repeated protamine sulphate	Start with 25–50mg, then dose by clinical response
Therapeutic use in pregnancy	? Repeated anti-Xa assays required
Around 3% bone loss in normal pregnancy	Around 5% bone loss with LMWH in pregnancy

APTT, Activated partial thromboplastin time.

lant function. Two classes of heparin are used clinically: unfractionated heparin (UFH), which contains a mixture of molecular weights, and the fractionated low-molecular-weight heparins (LMWH: see Table 5.3). Binding of UFH to antithrombin changes the conformational structure of antithrombin, resulting in a 1000-fold increase in its ability to inactivate factor (F) Xa and FIIa. The smaller fragments contained in LMWH preferentially bind the antithrombin–FXa complex.

The heparins currently available are inactive orally and have to given by an intravenous or subcutaneous route. The half-life of intravenous UFH is variable, but can be as short as 30–45 minutes. The therapeutic level of UFH can be assessed by an activated partial thromboplastin time (APTT or PTT: see Chapter 1). This is achieved by determining a ratio of the APTT in the patient sample to the APTT of a normal pooled plasma: this gives a therapeutic range of 1.5–2.5. Unlike warfarin, there is no internationally accepted standardized ratio. Indeed, when used in pregnancy, it must be remembered that the APTT may be shortened in pregnancy (as a result of an increase in the levels of key proteins such as FVIIIc, fibrinogen and the heparin-binding proteins), giving the impression of heparin resistance. When given subcutaneously, UFHs have a half-life of around 1.5 hours, and dose monitoring can be achieved by mid-interval APTT assessment (4–6 hours after dosing). The rate of major bleeding in pregnancies treated with UFH is 2%, which is consistent with the bleeding risk associated with both UFH and warfarin therapy in non-pregnant subjects treated for DVT. Furthermore it should be noted that dose-adjusted subcutaneous UFH can cause a persistent anticoagulant effect up to 28 hours after the last injection, which could be problematic at the time of delivery. However, the mechanism for this effect is unclear.

LMWHs are given subcutaneously and have more predictable kinetics and >90% bioavailability. This results in a half-life of 4–6 hours, which allows once, or twice, a day dosing, and monitoring is seldom required. The APTT is insensitive to the presence of LMWH (even when present in excess) and is likely to remain within reference limits. If monitoring of these drugs is needed, this can be achieved by assessment of the effect of the LMWH on the inactivation of coagulation FXa (an anti-Xa assay).

Reversal of intravenous UFH can be achieved by protamine sulfate injection: the amount to be given can be titrated to the predicted residual amount of UFH in the circulation, which routinely results in a protamine dose of 25–50mg. The downside of the long half-life of LMWHs is the difficulty in reversing their effect if bleeding occurs, or an excess dose is given accidentally. Protamine will inhibit only the LMWH currently in the circulation. In these circumstances, if bleeding is ongoing, it has been suggested that further protamine dosing should be determined by clinical response alone, although an initial anti-Xa assessment is often carried out in these circumstances. The anti-Xa level does not, however, predict bleeding, and the frequent monitoring which would be required to determine protamine dosing is often impractical. This problem can be significant, as an excess of protamine can also act as an anticoagulant.

Heparin-induced thrombocytopenia

There are two types of thrombocytopenia associated with heparin (see also Chapter 8). The first is non-immune heparin-induced thrombocytopenia (HIT), which is sometimes less accurately described as Type 1 HIT. This is a benign non-immune condition that results in a mild degree of thrombocytopenia, which appears to be due to a direct effect of heparin on the platelet membrane and is not associated with clinical symptoms, or thrombosis.

The more important type of thrombocytopenia associated with heparin is Type 2 HIT, also known as HIT thrombosis syndrome (HITTS), reflecting the clinical expression of the syndrome with thrombosis as well as thrombocytopenia. This immune condition arises from the development of specific heparin-dependent immunoglobulin (IgG) antibodies against the platelet factor (PF) 4–heparin complex. It commonly has its onset 5–14 days after the commencement of therapy, although it can occur after a brief exposure if there has been prior heparin exposure within the previous 3 months. This leads to platelet activation, generation of pro-coagulant microparticles from the platelet membrane and platelet consumption. Platelet levels can fall to a median of around $60 \times 10^9/l$, but levels $<20 \times 10^9/l$ are encountered in 10–15% of cases. Furthermore, a significant fall which does not result in a level less than the lower limit of the reference range can still be consistent with the diagnosis of Type 2 HIT. In addition to platelet consumption, Type 2 HIT is also associated with thrombin generation. This occurs via the generation of TF on endothelial cells activated by HIT antibodies binding to PF4 found on endothelial heparan sulfate, as well as increased expression of TF on monocytes upon activation by HIT antibodies. Clinically severe arterial or venous thrombotic complications can ensue. In 5–10% of subjects there may be venous thromboembolism, but myocardial infarction, limb ischemia, mesenteric artery thrombosis and cerebrovascular thrombosis also occur. The occurrence of thrombosis in affected patients is associated with a significant mortality. Interestingly, despite the thromboctyopenia, petechiae are absent, but skin reactions at injection sites and systemic inflammatory reactions can also occur. Thus, if a patient develops a skin reaction whilst on heparin it is prudent to monitor the platelet count for HIT.

The incidence of HIT has been estimated at 2.7% with UFH, and there is anecdotal evidence that HIT also occurs with LMWH, although the incidence is less easy to define. The incidence of HIT with LMWHs could be as low as 0% and the overall relative risk is likely to be at least 8-fold greater with UFH than LMWH. This is likely to relate to the heparin polysaccharide chain length, which needs to be at least 12–14 polysaccharides long to form an HIT antigen with PF4. The risk of both HIT and thrombosis varies with the patient type, the duration of use and the type of heparin. With UFH, cardiac surgery patients are most at risk of developing antibodies (around 50%), but few (<5% of those who become antibody positive) develop HIT, while orthopedic surgical patients have a lower rate of antibody development (15%), but as many as one third will go on to develop

HIT. It is important to note that HIT does not always lead to a clinical thrombotic event. Indeed, in cardiac surgery with UFH, 1% or less will develop a thrombotic problem.

There are occasional reports of thrombocytopenia or heparin-dependent platelet-activating antibodies in pregnant patients treated with LMWH. However, even in pregnant patients diagnosed with HIT associated with LMWH, there is often a previous sensitization or HIT episode related to UFH exposure. In general terms, medical and obstetric patients are considered least at risk, and recent recommendations do not consider that routine monitoring of the platelet count is required with LMWH use in pregnancy (the risk with LMWH in pregnancy is considered to be <0.1%). Thus, platelet count monitoring should be restricted to special situations (see Table 5.4).

HIT is a clinicopathologic syndrome, although the diagnosis is principally a clinical one, supported by the detection of serologic factors. Key factors to con-

Table 5.4 – Heparin-induced thrombocytopenia (HIT)

Those at risk	UFH > LMWH 5+ days treatment Previous HIT/previous UFH exposure
Consider platelet monitoring if:	On LMWH with previous exposure to UFH within 3 months UFH used prior to LMWH UFH is used for treatment or prevention of thrombosis A systemic reaction after intravenous UFH occurs A cutaneous reaction to UFH/LMWH occurs
Consider HIT diagnosis if:	An unexpected fall in platelet count occurs A new thrombotic problem has occurred A skin reaction is accompanied by thrombocytopenia Thrombocytopenia cannot be attributed to an established/alternative illness (including major VTE) Heparin is used in intravenous flushes or dialysis +/– HIT antibodies detected
Thrombosis types	MI, VTE, ArtT
Cross-reaction	LMWH may cross-react with UFH LMWH may cross-react with each other Danaparoid can also cross-react with heparin
Action	Stop all exposure to heparin Change to danaparoid/ hirudin/ ?warfarin Avoid platelet transfusions

ArtT, Arterial thrombisis; LMWH, Low-moleclular-weight heparin; MI, Myocardial infarction; UFH, Unfractionated heparin; VTE, Venous thromboembolism.

sider in making the diagnosis are shown in Table 5.4. HIT antibodies can be detected by either platelet-activation (functional) assays or by antigen assays directed against the heparin–PF4 complex. The diagnostic specificity of a sensitive washed platelet activation functional assay is greater than that of an antigen assay. The diagnosis of HIT is made when there is an otherwise unexplained fall in the platelet count (usually >50%, even if the platelet count remains >150×10^9/l), when there are skin lesions at heparin injection sites, or when an acute systemic reaction such as cardiorespiratory distress after intravenous heparin administration has occurred. The diagnosis is supported by the detection of HIT antibodies, but can be made even when there is a failure to confirm the presence of such antibodies. HIT antibody seroconversion on its own (i.e. without thrombocytopenia or other clinical sequelae) is not, however, considered sufficient to constitute a diagnosis of HIT.

Treatment centers on the discontinuation of any heparin preparation and the use of alternative thrombin inhibitors, usually in therapeutic doses. These alternatives include: the heparinoid, danaparoid; recombinant hirudin; and the direct thrombin inhibitor argatroban. Fondaparinux has also been employed in this context. While warfarin is best for chronic therapy, it should be avoided in the acute stage, as (noted above) it may result in a precipitous fall in the endogenous vitamin K-dependent anticoagulant protein S. This may result in skin necrosis and venous limb gangrene: those patients with protein C, protein S or antithrombin deficiency, or FV Leiden carriage are perhaps most at risk. Warfarin should therefore be delayed until the platelet count is >100×10^9/l and the HIT is resolving with the use of other antithrombotic agents. Adjunctive treatments that have been employed in the management of HIT include: embolectomy; plasmapheresis; thrombolysis; and high-dose intravenous normal immunoglobulin (to inhibit the antibody-mediated platelet activation). It should be noted that platelet component therapy should be avoided in HIT patients, as it is thought that this may increase platelet consumption and precipitate thrombosis.

UFH versus LMWH in pregnancy

Both UFH and LMWH have been used extensively in pregnancy. Heparins do not cross the placenta or enter breast milk, and no significant association with fetal disorders has been found. However, heparins have been linked to an increased maternal risk of osteoporosis, allergic reactions, HIT and hemorrhagic complications.

Osteoporosis

Of all the potential complications of heparin, perhaps the side effect that concerns obstetricians most is osteoporosis. Pregnancy itself is associated with a reduction in bone mineral density of the order of 3%. With prolonged UFH use, >30% of women on UFH will lose significant (>10%) bone mass. This is related to the dose and duration of therapy, and is more common with prolonged high-dose treatment. However, problems have been reported with doses as low as 15 000 day and with therapy given for only 7 weeks. In one study of long-term prophylactic UFH therapy in pregnancy, a 2.2% incidence of vertebral fractures was reported. Although, in another study, spinal fractures were reported in as many as 15% of patients receiving UFH at a dose of 10 000IU twice daily for a period of 3–6 months.

Experimental model and animal studies provide some insight into the mechanism of heparin-induced osteoporosis. A dose-dependent decrease in cancellous bone in the femur (resulting from decreased bone formation and increased bone resorption) occurs in animals treated with UFH for 1 month. In one animal study, UFH resulted in a 30% loss in cancellous bone during the first month of treatment. In this study, heparin was shown to accumulate in the bone and was retained there for at least a further 1 month after the cessation of therapy. This prolonged accumulation would suggest that heparin-induced osteoporosis may not be rapidly reversible.

LMWH carry a substantially lower risk of osteoporosis than UFH. In one study of non-pregnant venous thromboembolism (VTE) patients treated for 3–6 months, only 2.5% of subjects receiving LMWH experienced a vertebral fracture compared to 15% in the UFH group. One randomized trial of LMWH versus UFH in pregnancy measured bone mineral density in the lumbar spine for up to 3 years after delivery. In this study, bone density did not differ between healthy controls and the dalteparin group, but was significantly lower in the UFH group when compared to both controls and dalteparin-treated women. Multiple logistic regression found that the type of heparin therapy was the only independent factor associated with reduced bone mass. This is consistent with several observational pregnancy studies that have shown no difference in lumbar spine density in subjects on prolonged LMWH therapy and no greater bone loss than that which occurs in pregnancy naturally. In a review of LMWH (largely enoxaparin and dalteparin) therapy in over 2500 pregnancies, only one case of heparin-induced ostepenia with fracture (vertebral) was reported in a woman who had received a high dose (15 000IU/day) of dalteparin for a total of 36 weeks. Recently, however, three cases of osteoporotic fractures in association with tinzaparin use in pregnancy in one center have been reported. Whether this finding is causally related to tinzaparin (as additional therapies and underlying problems can also influence the development of osteoporosis) and whether this risk applies to other LMWH is unclear. In any event, the risk associated with LMWH remains very low in comparison to UFH. This difference between UFH and LMWH is consistent with animal studies, which show greater cancellous bone loss with UFH than LMWH.

Bleeding risk

LMWH appear to carry a lower risk of bleeding than UFH: severe bleeding problems have not been attributed to either treatment or prophylactic-dose LMWH during pregnancy. Furthermore, LMWH have not been associated with an increased risk of severe peripartum bleeding, with an observed rate of around 2%. This, in most cases, is linked to a primary obstetric cause, such as uterine atony or vaginal laceration, although it is possible that any such blood loss may be exacerbated by the presence of LMWH.

Antithrombotic efficacy

The effectiveness of LMWH in the management of thrombotic conditions in pregnancy is supported by the low VTE recurrence rate (just over 1%) reported during treatment in both large cohort studies and systematic reviews. This compares favorably with the recurrence rates of 5–8% reported in trials of non-pregnant patients treated with either LMWH or UFH (followed by coumarin therapy) after 3–6 month follow-up. LMWH thromboprophylaxis is also associated with a VTE rate of <1%.

Fetal outcome

With regard to fetal outcome, in general terms, the evidence supports a beneficial effect of LMWH on pregnancy loss rates. The successful pregnancy rate, reported in women receiving LMWH for previous adverse pregnancy outcomes (such as recurrent fetal loss), is >80%. This rate is consistent with that found in randomized trials of antithrombotic therapy (UFH or LMWH) in women with previous pregnancy loss associated with antiphospholipid syndrome or heritable thrombophilia, where such intervention resulted in a significant improvement in pregnancy outcome.

Kinetics and allergy

The half-life of LMWH is reduced in pregnancy due to the physiological increase in renal blood flow and glomerular filtration rate. Although allergic skin reactions occur in 1–2% of patients on LMWH, this risk is less than that with UFH and, as noted above, LMWH also carry a lesser risk of HIT. Thus, given their effectiveness, ease of use, safety for mother and fetus, and reliable kinetics, LMWH are, at present, the anticoagulants of choice in pregnancy.

Danaparoid

Danaparoid is a heparinoid (a mixture of heparan, dermatan and chondroitin sulfates), that inactivates FXa and FIIa. It has a relatively long half-life of 25 hours in non-pregnant subjects. Danaparoid has been used successfully in pregnancy-associated HIT and, out-with pregnancy, danaparoid is successful in >90% of cases. However, a positive cross-reaction can occur in 15% of cases of HIT. Danaparoid is also useful in pregnant patients with an allergy to LMWH. The thromboprophylactic dose for an average pregnant patient is 750IU given twice daily by subcutaneous injection. At a prophylactic dose, it has no effect on platelet function and should not be associated with excess blood loss at delivery. When a therapeutic dose is required, danaparoid can be monitored by an anti-Xa assay using a danaparoid control. The recommended dosing with danaparoid for HIT outwith pregnancy is an intravenous bolus of 2250IU, followed by an intravenous infusion at 400IU/hour for 4 hours, then 300IU/hour for 4 hours, then 200IU/hour adjusted by anti-Xa levels. It does not cross the placenta and although it is not yet clear whether it crosses the breast, this appears unlikely, as no anti-Xa activity occurs in breast milk. In any event, it should be destroyed in the infant GI tract. It is exclusively excreted by the kidney and should be used with extreme caution in subjects with renal failure.

Direct thrombin inhibitors

Thrombin inhibitors are potent inhibitors of both free and clot-bound thrombin, which do not cross-react with HIT antibodies and have little, or no, effect on related serine proteases.

Lepirudin

Lepirudin, a recombinant hirudin (hirudin is derived from the medicinal leech *Hirudo medicinalis*), binds tightly to thrombin with slow dissociation, making it effectively an irreversible inhibitor. There is very little information on its use in pregnancy, but it may have a role as an alternative to danaparoid in the management of pregnancy-related HIT. The dose used for HIT is an initial infusion of 0.15mg/kg/hour intravenously, with the aim to achieve a target APTT of 1.5–2.0 times either the patient's baseline APTT, or the mean of APTT laboratory reference range. It has a relatively short half-life of about 80 minutes and is renally excreted. At higher doses the ecarin clotting time has a more linear correlation with plasma hirudin levels and may be more useful for monitoring. In animal studies, hirudin has low placental transit and it does not appear to cross the breast. When considering the use of hirudin, it should be borne in mind that it currently has no antidote and it should be used with caution in those with renal impairment. In practice, the use of hirudin should be limited to those subjects where the HIT antibody is shown to cross-react with danaparoid, or in those who have a cutaneous allergy to danaparoid. There is a high rate of antibody development to hirudin of 40–60% and anaphylaxis can occur, although this is rare.

Argatroban

Argatroban is a synthetic thrombin inhibitor derived from L-arginine. It binds tightly, yet reversibly, to thrombin. Individuals receiving prolonged, or repeated, administration show no generation of antibodies and no enhancement or suppression of the anticoagulant response. It is metabolized in the liver and its effect can be monitored with the APTT (aiming to achieve 1.5–3 times control values). Its action is quickly reversed by stopping the infusion (<60 minutes), but clearance is reduced 3–4-fold if there is moderate hepatic impairment. It is used in the treatment of HIT where its effectiveness is clearly demonstrated. In this situation the recommended dose is an initial infusion rate of 2µg/kg/minute, with no initial bolus required. There is no significant experience of the use of this agent in pregnancy.

Aspirin

Aspirin irreversibly inhibits (through acetylation) cyclo-oxygenase, which is pivotal in the generation of thromboxane A_2 in the platelet. The effect of aspirin lasts between 7 and 10 days, as restoration of platelet function requires new platelet synthesis. Aspirin only partially inhibits adenosine diphosphate (ADP) and collagen-induced platelet activation, and has no effect on thrombin-mediated platelet activation. Aspirin may be as effective as an antithrombotic agent at modest doses (75mg/day) as it is at higher doses (1200mg/day). The principal side effects of aspirin are bleeding and idiosyncratic or allergic reactions. In children, ingestion of aspirin has been associated with Reye's syndrome.

Aspirin has been widely assessed for the prevention of pregnancy-related complications such as intrauterine growth restriction and pre-eclampsia. The use of low dose aspirin (60–75mg/day) to prevent pre-eclampsia is based upon the rationale that pre-eclampsia is associated with alterations in the production of prostacyclin and thromboxane, secondary to activation of the clotting system and changes in platelet function. A recent meta-analysis reported on 42 randomized trials involving over 32 000 women comparing antiplatelet agents to placebo or no treatment. Trials were subgrouped by maternal risk. Taking the cohort as a whole, there was a 15% reduction (relative risk 0.85, 95% confidence interval (CI) 0.78–0.92) in the risk of pre-eclampsia associated with the use of antiplatelet agents. These assessments have shown that low-dose aspirin (around 75mg/day) appears safe for use in pregnant women. At higher doses (>150mg/day) its safety, especially in the first trimester, is controversial.

Although aspirin has been shown to reduce the risk of venous thrombosis in the context of orthopedic surgery, its role in the context of pregnancy-related thrombosis is not yet defined. However, it does not appear to offer the same level of protection as UFH or LMWH for thromboprophylaxis. When aspirin has been used as a substitute to coumarins (in subjects with mechanical heart valves), as would be expected, it confers insufficient anticoagulation and results in an unacceptable (and often fatal) 25% incidence of systemic embolism and 4% incidence of valve thrombosis, although it appears safe from a fetal perspective.

Aspirin has a role in combination with other therapies, particularly in combination with LMWH, in the antiphospholipid syndrome. It is also of value where specific antiplatelet therapy is required in pregnancy, such as in women with a previous cerebral ischemia of arterial origin, ischemic heart disease or essential thrombocythemia, or when other anticoagulant therapies are unsuitable.

The salicylates, including aspirin, are excreted at low doses in breast milk, with <10% reaching the nursing infant. Although this could cause drug accumulation in the fetus, maternal doses of <100mg/day are considered safe as regards infant bleeding. Overall, as there is a risk that high-dose maternal aspirin could lead to bleeding in the infant, and because of a theoretical risk of Reye's syndrome, aspirin is not advised for nursing mothers in a number of countries.

Dextran

Dextran has been used for peripartum thromboprophylaxis, particularly during Cesarean section. It does, however, carry a significant risk of anaphylactic and anaphylactoid reactions, which have been associated with uterine hypertonus, profound fetal distress, and a high incidence of fetal death or profound neurological damage. Thus, dextran for thromboprophylaxis should be avoided prior to delivery.

New anticoagulant therapies

There are a number of new anticoagulants in development. These include substances aimed at the onset of coagulation, such as tissue factor pathway inhibitors, to drugs aimed at the downregulation of thrombin generation. In addition, there is work ongoing to develop an orally active heparin derivative. Of the drugs in development, two classes have completed a number of clinical trials and may soon achieve licences for use in non-pregnant subjects. These are the synthetic pentassaccharides fonduparinux and idraparinux (which, like heparin, inactivate FXa by binding to antithrombin), and the direct thrombin inhibitor melagatran, which is given orally (as its pro-drug, ximelagatran).

Fondaparinux and Idraparinux

Fondaparinux binds to antithrombin, which results in a 300-fold increase in antithrombin activity against FXa. It has a half-life of around 17 hours after subcutaneous injection and has been shown to be efficacious in the prevention of VTE after orthopedic surgery. It has been used in pregnancy where women developed skin reactions to LMWH. Fondaparinux appears to pass the placental barrier in vivo (in contrast to in vitro where no transfer is found), resulting in measurable anti-FXa activity in umbilical cord blood. However, the concentration of fondaparinux in umbilical cord blood appears to be well below the concentration required for effective anticoagulation. Nonetheless, because of this, the availability of alternative therapies, and limited safety data, fondaparinux should be avoided at present, or its use limited to those for whom there are no therapeutic alternatives. Idraparinux is another synthetic pentassaccharide which also leads to FXa inhibition, but has a prolonged half-life (80 hours), which could allow once weekly dosing. There are currently no data on its use in pregnancy. Protamine sulfate has no action on these drugs, but two studies have shown that recombinant FVIIa (rFVIIa) may be able to reverse the biochemical changes induced by these pentassaccharides in healthy volunteers. In future, heparinases may also have a role in their inactivation.

Ximelagatran

Ximelagatran is the prodrug of melagatran, which is an active site-directed thrombin inhibitor. Ximelagatran is well absorbed from the gut and has a plasma half-life of 3–4 hours, allowing it to be administered twice daily. Thus, it has the potential of being an alternative oral anticoagulant to warfarin. It may require a dose adjustment when there is renal impairment, and in 6% of subjects a mild rise in transaminases has been noted, although more severe reactions have also occurred. This has led to concerns for the safety of this agent and it remains unlicensed in both the USA and Europe at present. It appears most likely that ximelagatran will have a role in the prophylaxis of atrial fibrillation in the first instance. At present, however, there is insufficient information on the safety of this class of compounds in those who are pregnant or breastfeeding.

CHAPTER 6
Management of thrombotic disorders

Pregnancy places a substantial demand on the cardiovascular system. With increasing gestation there is a 30–50% increase in cardiac output, which is accompanied by an increase in prothrombotic coagulation factors, a decrease in some natural anticoagulants and an alteration in systemic fibrinolysis. This preparation for the hemostatic challenge of delivery poses a particular threat to those women at risk of thrombosis.

More and more, obstetricians and hematologists are faced with the management of pregnant subjects who have risk factors for either arterial or venous thrombosis. This most commonly includes those with a previous thrombosis or those with prosthetic heart valves, but there is an evolving awareness of genetic and acquired risk factors that may identify those at particular risk of vascular occlusion, not only in pregnancy but also in later life.

Arterial thrombosis in pregnancy

Acute arterial occlusion during pregnancy is very rare and evidence for its management is based upon case reports and small case series, with most data extrapolated from non-pregnant subjects. More relevant to routine care, is the prevention of disease in those at risk and minimizing the potential harm of anticoagulants to the mother and the fetus. Recently, there has also been the suggestion that women with risk factors for arterial thrombosis are also at higher risk of other pregnancy complications, such as pre-eclampsia, growth restriction and fetal loss.

Risk factors for arterial disease in pregnancy

Arterial occlusion is usually the end result of a prolonged process that terminates in the rupture of an atherosclerotic plaque with intramural thrombotic occlusion, and a number of common factors are recognized as risks for arterial disease (see Table 6.1). Of these, those that are relevant in women of childbearing age include hypercholesterolemia, smoking, hypertension, diabetes mellitus, obesity, low socio-economic status and a family history of ischemic heart disease. A number of rarer systemic disorders are also associated with an increased risk of vascular occlusion during pregnancy: these include essential thrombocythemia,

Table 6.1 – Risk factors for arterial thrombosis in young women

Hypercholesterolemia
Family history of ischemic heart disease
Smoking
Hypertension
Diabetes mellitus
Obesity
Essential thrombocythemia
Polcythemia rubra vera
Sickle-cell disease
Prosthetic heart valve
Mitral stenosis and atrial fibrillation
Mitral bioprothesis and atrial fibrillation
Mechanical mitral valve
Antiphospholipid syndrome
? Smoking with Factor V Leiden or prothrombin 20210A
Hyperhomocysteinemia
Cocaine
Ergot
?Marijuana
Previous cerebral ischemia of arterial origin
Previous myocardial infarction
Hypotension
Pre-eclampsia

primary polycythemia and paroxysmal nocturnal hemoglobinuria (see Chapter 3). In addition, those with prosthetic heart valves, or a prior history of arterial occlusion, are also at higher risk of arterial occlusion during pregnancy. Other, more intriguing, risks for arterial occlusion that may have a bearing in the pregnancy age group include cocaine and marijuana use. There is also the historical consideration that the ergot derivatives used in the management of postpartum hemorrhage may also be associated with an increased risk of arterial occlusion.

Recently, there has been interest in the possible risk resulting from the combination of acquired risk factors and single gene defects (see Chapter 7). These include: elevated plasma factor (F) VIIIc levels (resulting from the interaction of blood groups with the acute phase response); hyperhomocysteinemia (due to the combination of hematinic deficiency and enzyme defects in the homocysteine–methionine pathway); acquired activated protein C resistance (due to a combination of arterial and venous thrombotic risk factors) and; the antiphospholipid syndrome. Indeed, a small number of studies have suggested that there may also be a link between either the prothrombin G20210A or FV Leiden mutations and arterial disease in young female smokers. This remains disputed, but, if confirmed, will contrast with more severe heritable thrombophilias, such as antithrombin, or protein C or S deficiency, where there has never been convincing evidence of a link with arterial thrombosis.

Pregnancy with valvular heart disease or prosthetic heart valves

Valvular heart disease results from either congenital cardiac disorders or rheumatic heart disease. Rheumatic disease most commonly affects the mitral valve and may result in stenosis, or incompetence. Indeed, previously undiagnosed mitral stenosis may present for the first time in pregnancy with thromboembolism, due to the onset of atrial fibrillation. In such cases, atrial fibrillation may be induced by the change in cardiac output and cardiac pressures that accompany normal gestation. Overall, the risk of thromboembolism from a mitral stenosis has been estimated at <4.5%/annum when there is sinus rhythm, although the risk is likely to be around 10 times higher at the onset of atrial fibrillation.

Pregnancy in a woman with a prosthetic mechanical heart valve is not a benign process. Overall, mechanical valves carry a 1–4% risk of maternal mortality, mainly arising from complications of valve thrombosis. Inadequate anticoagulation increases the risk of thromboembolism, such that subjects with mechanical prosthetic valves require full anticoagulation throughout pregnancy. This may be especially the case when the patient has an older valve type (such as Starr-Edwards or Bjork-Shiley) and atrial fibrillation, and where the valve is in the mitral position.

Patients with bioprosthetic valves do not usually require anticoagulation in pregnancy, and those subjects with satisfactory cardiovascular adaptation have a good fetal outcome. There is, however, concern that pregnancy may result in accelerated calcification of bioprosthetic valves. In one retrospective audit, around 35% of pregnancies in subjects with bioprosthetic valves had sufficient deterioration in valve function during the pregnancy such that replacement was required during, or soon after, pregnancy. However, this effect of pregnancy on the valve has not been confirmed in a further study of the long-term experience of such valves where a history of pregnancy was not associated with a higher risk of valve failure.

Management of valvular heart disease or prosthetic heart valves in pregnancy

Given the potential risk of thromboembolism associated with mitral valve stenosis, anticoagulant prophylaxis may be appropriate during pregnancy in those women with additional risk factors such as atrial fibrillation or heart failure. As noted above, there is not usually a requirement for anticoagulation in women with bioprosthetic valves unless they have additional risk factors.

The management of pregnancy in women with mechanical prosthetic valves remains controversial, as there are few controlled trials to guide optimal antithrombotic therapy. In addition, the balance of risk between the potential fetal and maternal complications with the currently available therapies – warfarin and heparin (see Chapter 5) – is also unknown. In particular, in view of the concerns with oral coumarin therapy, there is a need to find alternative strategies that are will be safe for both the mother and the fetus.

A recent review of maternal and fetal outcomes in women with prosthetic heart valves reported that commonly used anticoagulant regimes were: (1) use of coumarin throughout pregnancy; (2) replacement of coumarin with unfractionated heparin (UFH) from 6 to 12 weeks gestation; and (3) UFH use throughout pregnancy. Overall, fetal wastage was 33.6% in the first group, 26.5% in the second and 19.6% in the third. In the coumarin regimes, heparin was used at term to avoid delivery with an anticoagulated mother and fetus. Coumarin embryopathy occurred in 6.4% of live births where a coumarin was used through pregnancy: this was eliminated if heparin was substituted by 6 weeks gestation.

In this review (see Table 6.2), coumarin use through pregnancy was associated with a lower risk of thromboembolic problems (3.9%) when compared with pregnancies where heparin was substituted for the coumarin. UFH used between 6 and 12 weeks gestation was associated with a risk of valve thrombosis of 9.2%, and UFH used throughout pregnancy was associated with a 25% rate of valve thrombosis with adjusted-dose heparin and a 60% rate with low-dose UFH. However, the numbers of patients exposed to UFH included in the review was modest. In addition, many thromboembolic events were associated with an inadequate heparin dosage. Moreover, modern bi-leaflet valves are substantially less thrombogenic than earlier mechanical valves such as the Bjork-Shiley and Starr-Edwards valves, which were predominant in most of the work reviewed. These limitations make it difficult to extrapolate early work directly to contemporary practice with modern valves and well-controlled anticoagulation with UFH (or indeed low-molecular-weight heparin (LMWH)) with regard to thrombotic risk.

Table 6.2 – Maternal outcomes from women with mechanical valves receiving anticoagulation

Anticoagulation schedule	Thromboembolism (%)	Death (%)
Coumarin/heparin	3.9	1.8
Heparin/coumarin/heparin	9.2*	4.2
Adjusted-dose heparin	25.0*	6.7
Low-dose heparin	60.0	40.0
No heparin or antiplatelet therapy alone	24.3	4.7

After Chan et al 2000.

*Up to 50% of complications occurred on low-dose heparin and others with inadequate dosing based on the activated partial thromboplastin time. There is a 2.5% incidence of severe bleeding at delivery and the rate with low-molecular-weight heparin is unclear with an estimate of 13%.

Thus, on the basis of the limited data available, coumarin appears more effective than UFH for thromboembolic prophylaxis in women with mechanical heart valves in pregnancy (Table 6.2), but UFH is associated with a better fetal outcome (see Table 6.3).

The situation is changing with the increasing use of LMWH in pregnant women with prosthetic heart valves, which has attractions over UFH in terms of monitoring and maternal side effects, although concerns still exist over how effective LMWH is for thrombrophylaxis in this situation. In a review of 67 pregnancies treated with LMWH in women with prosthetic valves, valve thrombosis occurred in seven cases, giving an incidence of 10.4% (95% confidence interval (CI), 3.1–17.7%) and a mortality rate of 1.49% (95% CI, 0.03–8.34%). The overall thromboembolic complication rate was 13.4% (9 in 67; 95% CI, 5.4–21.4%). However, eight of the nine patients with a thromboembolic complication had received a fixed dose of LMWH, and in two of these patients, a fixed low-dose of LMWH. In 42 pregnancies with anti-Xa levels monitored, only one thromboembolic complication occurred. The live birth rate was 89.5% (95% CI, 82.5–96.5%), the fetal wastage was 8.9% (95% CI, 2.1–15.7%) and there were no reported congenital anomalies. Thus, adjusted-dose LMWH (anti-Xa level at a minimum of 1.0IU/ml) compares favorably with UFH in this situation.

Because of the limited data, management remains controversial and several approaches remain acceptable, including substitution of LMWH for UFH. However, it is clearly critical to ensure adequate doses of UFH or LMWH. There is still a need for consensus among experts to systematically gather the best available evidence, identify unresolved issues and generate studies designed to answer these questions. Meanwhile, the American College of Chest Physicians (ACCP) recommends either adjusted-dose twice-daily LMWH throughout pregnancy, in doses adjusted either to keep a 4 hourly post-injection anti-Xa level at around 1.0–1.2IU/ml (preferably) or in doses adjusted by weight. Alternatively, aggres-

Table 6.3 – Fetal outcome in women with mechanical valves receiving anticoagulation

Treatment	Spontaneous miscarriage (%)	Congenital anomaly (%)	Fetal wastage (%)
Coumarin throughout, with/without heparin at term	24.8	6.4	33.6
Heparin in first trimester, then coumarin	24.8	3.5	26.5
Heparin throughout	9.8	3.4*	19.6

After Chan et al 2000

*None if heparin started before 6 weeks

Table 6.4 – Management of mechanical prosthetic valves

Option 1	Dose-adjust UFH, 12 hourly subcutaneous, throughout pregnancy
	Mid-interval APTT ≥ 2 × control or
	Anti-Xa 0.35–0.70IU/ml
Option 2	Dose-adjust (by weight) LMWH throughout pregnancy
	4 hour post-injection anti-Xa around 1.0IU/ml
Option 3	UFH or LMWH till 13th week
	Change to warfarin until mid-third trimester
	Restart UFH or LMWH until delivery
Option 4	Warfarin throughout pregnancy
	with substitution of UFH or LMWH in late third trimester for delivery

APTT, Activated partial thromboplastin time; LMWH, Low-molecular-weight heparin; UFH, Unfractionated heparin.

sive adjusted-dose UFH throughout pregnancy, i.e. administered subcutaneously, 12 hourly, in doses adjusted to keep the mid-interval activated partial thromboplastin time (APTT) at least twice control, or to attain an anti-Xa heparin level of 0.35–0.70IU/ml, can be used. One further option proposed is UFH or LMWH (as above) until the 13th week, with a change to warfarin until the middle of the third trimester, and then restarting UFH or LMWH (see Table 6.4). The ACCP also suggest the addition of low-dose aspirin.

Long-term oral anticoagulants should be resumed postpartum with all regimens, but there appears to be a significant risk of secondary postpartum hemorrhage when switching from therapeutic heparin to therapeutic coumarin soon after delivery, and so the present authors delay this switch for several days after delivery to minimize the risk whenever possible.

Cerebral ischemia of arterial origin (CIAO) in pregnancy

CIAO may result from atherosclerosis, from emboli of cardiac origin or from hypotension. There is also an association between arteritis or antiphospholipid syndrome and small-vessel brain disease. In published literature, there is a great variation in the estimate of risk of CIAO during pregnancy. This may be due to a lack of computerized tomography (CT) or magnetic resonance imaging (MRI) in early studies, or failure to distinguish venous from arterial cerebral thrombosis in some. Other studies are also compromised by their small sample size or referral bias. This results in a quoted risk of CIAO in pregnancy which varies from 1 in 5000 to 1 in 20000 pregnancies, with the latter figure suggesting that pregnancy may be associated with only a marginal risk when compared with non-pregnant subjects (at around 5 in 100000/women-years).

Most CIAO occur in the puerperium or the third trimester and, in >50% of cases there may be evidence of a major arterial occlusion. In a substantial number of cases, however, no evidence of major occlusion is found either at angiogram or post-mortem. A number of common risk factors relate to CIAO in pregnancy as they do in the non-pregnant. These include hypertension, smoking, pre-existing premature atherosclerosis and valvular heart disease. In pregnancy, eclampsia is also associated with small-vessel cerebral complications. CIAO is likely to be more common in older women, in those with sepsis and in those who have undergone Cesarean section delivery. However, in many studies, a clear distinction between ischemic and other cerebral events is not made. In addition, rarer causes – such as choriocarcinoma, paradoxical embolism, sickle-cell disease, lupus inhibitor-related thrombosis, ergot alkaloid usage and homocystinuria – have also been reported in the etiology of pregnancy-related CIAO.

Management of CIAO in pregnancy

The investigation and management of CIAO in pregnancy should follow national guidelines on the management of CIAO in non-pregnant subjects (see Table 6.5). This should include, as a minimum, CT or MRI imaging to locate the infarct and to determine if there is evidence of an associated cerebral hemorrhage.

CIAO may result in a fatal maternal outcome in 0–26% of cases. In one study, 13 recurrences were reported in the 5-year follow of a cohort of 373 women with a history of CIAO related to pregnancy. The majority of these were observed in relation to a subsequent pregnancy, with around a 2-fold higher risk associated with the puerperium when compared with the antepartum period. Interestingly, the overall outcome of subsequent pregnancies was similar to that expected in the general population.

Although there is no substantial evidence to support its use, low-dose aspirin therapy may be beneficial in the prevention of CIAO recurrence during pregnancy. In addition, the delivery should be managed to minimize the risk of venous and arterial thrombosis. In particular, a prolonged second stage of labor should be avoided and, if there is reduced mobility due to hemiplegia, there may be a requirement for LMWH thromboprophylaxis. It has also been suggested that those with a previously identified thrombophilic disorder may benefit from LMWH therapy in subsequent pregnancies, although the validity of this approach is not known.

Acute myocardial infarction in pregnancy

Acute myocardial infarction occurring during pregnancy may result in significant fetal and maternal morbidity. It is, however, a relatively rare event, which occurs in only 1 in 10 000 women. In general, most myocardial infarctions occur in multigravid women, and a cumulative maternal mortality rate of 21% has been reported.

Table 6.5 – Management of those with cerebral ischemia of arterial origin (CIAO) or myocardial infarction (MI) in pregnancy

CIAO	Previous	Low-dose aspirin	Yes
		Avoid long second stage	Yes
		VTE thromboprophylaxis	Yes
MI	Acute	Delay delivery for ≥2 weeks	Yes
		Thrombolytic therapy	?
		Low-dose aspirin	Yes
		High-dose aspirin	?
		LMWH	Yes
		Nitrates	Yes
		Beta-blockers	Yes
		Calcium-channel blockers	Yes
		Opiates	Yes
		Magnesium sulfate	Yes
		ACE inhibitors	No
		↓ Delivery stress	?Cesarian section
		VTE thromboprophylaxis	Yes
		Maternal death	Fetal delivery <15 minutes
	Previous	Assessment	Cause
			Current IHD
			Evidence of LVF

ACE, Angiotensin-converting enzyme; IHD, Ischaemic heart disease; LMWH, Low-molecular-weight heparin; LVF, Left ventricular function; VTE, Venous thromboembolism.

Although infarction may occur at any gestation, the majority of deaths occur at, or within 2 weeks of, the infarction, and often during labor or delivery. In subjects in whom a post-mortem was carried out, coronary atherosclerosis was evident in 43% of subjects and probable coronary thrombosis, without evidence of atherosclerotic disease, was evident in 21%. Atherosclerosis was more commonly found in subjects with an antipartum myocardial infarction than in those with a postpartum event. Dissection of the coronary artery was found in 16% of subjects and was more often associated with infarction in the puerperium. No detectable evidence of coronary occlusion was found in around 30% of antepartum and 75% of postpartum events. The absence of detectable occlusive disease may indicate a significant role of transient coronary artery spasm in these subjects.

It is likely that the prothrombotic changes in coagulation, which occur even in normal pregnancy, increase the risk for arterial thrombosis. These include an increase in coagulation factors and a reduction in the coagulation inhibitor protein S (although heritable protein S deficiency is not associated with adult arterial thrombosis). Furthermore, at delivery, an increase in coagulation may be induced by separation of the placenta, which is the principal source of tissue plasminogen activator (tPA) inhibitor. In cases of coronary dissection, the etiology remains unknown, but may relate to changes in arterial histology (such as alteration in elastic and reticular fibers, and mucopolysaccharide composition) which are a feature of normal gestation. Such changes may be compounded by pre-existing risk factors for coronary heart disease, as well as the increasing blood volume/heart rate, myocardial oxygen requirements, anemia and the reduction in diastolic blood pressure that are a feature of normal pregnancy.

Diagnosis and management of myocardial infarction in pregnancy

The diagnosis of myocardial infarction in pregnant women should be achieved in the same way as in non-pregnant subjects. The use of invasive or radiological techniques, however, requires an assessment of the balance of risks and benefits in each case. It is also recognized that electrocardiographic changes may be difficult to interpret during elective Cesarean section or delivery, and that tachycardia, atrial and ventricular ectopics are a feature of normal pregnancy.

Although the management of myocardial infarction in pregnancy is comparable with that of non-pregnant subjects, the presence of a viable fetus may influence the modalities of therapy used (Table 6.5). In particular, morphine sulfate crosses the placenta and may cause neonatal respiratory depression when given shortly before delivery, although in practice this does not usually cause a significant clinical problem. Currently, thrombolytic therapy is contraindicated in pregnancy due to the potential for teratogenesis. However, there is no evidence that streptokinase crosses the placenta in late pregnancy or, to a significant degree, during labor. Indeed, the majority of reports using streptokinase or tPA have shown a favorable fetal outcome, although maternal hemorrhage and an increased risk of pre-term delivery and fetal loss has been reported (see below).

As with the management of mechanical valves, heparin is the anticoagulant of choice in pregnancy. Aspirin therapy, at a low dose of ~150mg/day, appears safe in the second and third trimesters of pregnancy, and although aspirin is secreted in breast milk, this is in low concentrations. The safety of high-dose aspirin during pregnancy is not established. In general, the use of drugs such as nitrates, beta-blockers, calcium-channel blockers and magnesium sulfate are generally considered to be acceptable during pregnancy. However, angiotensin-converting enzyme (ACE) inhibitors are contraindicated, due to an increased risk of fetal morbidity and mortality.

If possible, delivery should be postponed until 2–3 weeks after the acute event, as labor and delivery may increase the risk of myocardial ischemia. There is, currently, no specific recommendation on the safest mode of delivery and an individual approach is required to minimize maternal cardiac workload. However, if the event occurs close to term, elective Cesarean section is likely to be the safest option for the mother, as this avoids the cardiovascular stress of labor and the possibility of an emergency Cesarean section, which carries a substantially greater risk of complications. There may also be a role for continuing LMWH, due to the increased risk of venous thrombosis that may occur as a consequence of cardiac failure, immobility or concurrent inflammation. There may be a requirement to avoid neuraxial anesthesia if a combination of aspirin and clopidogrel is used, as it may be associated with a more marked increase in the bleeding time than aspirin alone. When a maternal death has occurred there should be a rapid delivery if a viable fetus is to be secured.

The risk associated with future pregnancy is dependent on the etiology of the event, the presence of persisting myocardial ischemia and the degree of residual impairment of left ventricular function.

Venous thrombosis in pregnancy

As noted above, pregnancy is associated with hypercoagulability, venous stasis (from pelvic vein compression by the gravid uterus) and the vascular trauma induced by delivery. It is no surprise then, that in developed countries, venous thromboembolism (VTE) remains a major cause of maternal morbidity and mortality.

VTE occurs in <1 in 1000 deliveries, but may be 5–10 times more common in pregnancy than in non-pregnant women of the same age. In addition, those with a previous thrombosis have a 3.5-fold increased risk of recurrence in a future pregnancy, with a risk that has been estimated as falling between 0 and 13%. Not surprisingly, prospective studies produce the more conservative estimates of recurrence than retrospective analyses. A lower risk of antenatal recurrence has been observed when the first VTE is associated with a transient risk factor and there is no evidence of a thrombophilia disorder (2.4%), when compared with those with either an idiopathic VTE or evidence of thrombophilia (6%). The risk per day is higher in the first 6 weeks after delivery (the puerperium) than it is antepartum, with 40% of VTE occurring after discharge from hospital. However, VTE can occur in any trimester, and occurs in the left leg in around 90% of pregnancy-associated cases: a feature that may result from compression of the left iliac vein by the right iliac and ovarian arteries.

After a pregnancy-related deep-vein thrombosis (DVT) as many as 80% of subjects will experience post-phlebitic symptoms (swelling, skin discoloration, inflammation and skin ulceration), with around 20% of women required to use compression stockings up to 10 years after the event. As might be anticipated, the risk of post-phlebitic symptoms is 2–3 times more likely in those presenting with a DVT than in those presenting with pulmonary thromboembolism (PTE).

DVT is accompanied by PTE in around 16% of cases, and this is the major source of mortality. Although the maternal mortality associated with PTE has reduced in recent years in developed countries, the rate is still of the order of around 2/million deliveries, with a higher rate in older women.

Diagnosis of VTE in pregnancy

It is likely that a clinical suspicion of DVT in pregnancy will be confirmed radiologically on only 10% of occasions when compared with 25% of non-pregnant subjects. Similarly, only 1.8% of suspected PTE in pregnancy have a high probability ventilation/perfusion (V/Q) scan, when compared with <35% of non-pregnant subjects where the clinical suspicion of PTE can be confirmed by objective diagnostic techniques. This need for an objective diagnosis is particularly important in pregnancy, as features such as leg edema and breathlessness are not uncommon. However, the requirement for a definitive diagnosis needs to be balanced with the need to minimize the radiation exposure to the mother and the fetus that may result from investigations such as CT, angiography, ventilation-perfusion scanning or venography.

Clinically, the patient with a VTE may observe unilateral leg swelling and pain, or the unexpected onset of breathlessness or chest pain. The use of the pre-test probability assessments (a history of VTE, D-dimer assessment etc), which are used in non-pregnant subjects to guide investigations, are also important in pregnancy, but are unlikely to have the same sensitivity or specificity.

DVT

The absence of elevated D-dimer levels (detected by enzyme-linked immunosorbent assay (ELISA) or whole blood agglutination assay) is useful to exclude VTE in non-pregnant subjects, where they have a high negative predictive value. As discussed in Chapter 1, elevated D-dimers are seen in around 50% of females in the first trimester, and may be universal in later pregnancy and the puerperium. On account of this, their ability to exclude VTE in pregnancy is not yet reliable. Although a 'normal' result may be helpful, D-dimer results in pregnancy do not remove the need for an objective diagnosis.

Although contrast venography is the gold-standard investigation for DVT diagnosis, compression ultrasound assessment is more likely to be used as the initial assessment. Ultrasound has a high sensitivity and specificity for proximal thrombosis in non-pregnant subjects, but has its greatest utility when used between the inguinal ligament and the bifurcation of the popliteal vein. If, on compression, the venous lumen collapses then there is unlikely to be thrombus present. When there is the possibility of an isolated iliac or calf DVT, compression ultrasound may be of less value in the exclusion of disease. In general, if there is a clinical suspicion, treatment should be started and ultrasound scanning of the lower limbs should be performed. If the scan is negative, and there is a low clinical suspicion, then treatment can be stopped. If, despite a negative scan, there is still a high clinical suspicion then treatment should be continued for 7 days and the scan should be repeated. When there is a suspicion of isolated calf disease, serial ultrasound assessment over the next 7–14 days, without treatment, has been proposed by some. This proposal is based upon the low risk of extension to popliteal and femoral vessels (of the order of 20–25%), and the low risk of embolization of isolated calf DVT, although the general applicability of this approach is not clear. There may also be a problem in the diagnosis of an isolated iliac thrombosis in pregnancy, as there may be difficulty in assessing the vein as it passes behind the pregnant uterus. This is, thankfully, an uncommon diagnostic problem and requires an individual approach to minimize the risk of fetal radiation exposure from venography or CT scanning.

As a guide, bilateral venography may result in fetal exposure of around 0.6rad without abdominal shielding, although more limited venography will markedly reduce exposure (perhaps to <0.05rad). It is thought that in utero exposure to <5rad does not result in fetal loss or congenital abnormality, but may be associated with a 2-fold increase in the risk of childhood malignancy. An alternative technique may be MRI, which appears to give no immediate problems, but its long-term effects on the fetus are unknown.

PTE

Patients with acute PTE in pregnancy often present with dysponea, but wheeze, unexplained fever, pleuritc pain, as well as central chest pain, cyanosis and collapse (associated with more massive thrombosis) may all be presenting features. In such patients, other potential diagnoses such as infection, effusion and pneumothorax, should be excluded by X-ray. Electrocardiogram (ECG) analysis does not produce a sufficiently specific pattern to diagnose PTE, and blood gas analysis interpretation is complicated by the presence of pregnancy-related respiratory alkalosis. The sampling procedure itself may also result in bleeding from the puncture site. Overall, blood gas analysis is probably not warranted in the routine diagnosis or exclusion of PTE in pregnancy. Indeed, X-ray examinations, blood gas analysis and ECG are, on their own, insufficient to exclude or diagnose PTE.

To investigate PTE in pregnancy, one potential strategy is to investigate the lower limbs for evidence of DVT by compression ultrasound. If the results are positive, treat the patient with a presumptive diagnosis of PTE.

When there is no alternative diagnosis that accounts for the symptoms and signs, and there is no evidence of a peripheral DVT, V/Q scanning should be performed. As this may result in fetal exposure of <0.5rad, useful information can be obtained from a perfusion scan alone in some cases. Avoidance of the ventilation scan can reduce the fetal exposure to <0.01rad. A positive result will, however, require a ventilation scan to exclude conditions such as pneumonia.

As in non-pregnant subjects, a V/Q scan will lead to three possible outcomes: a high probability of PTE (a large ventilation/perfusion mismatch); an intermediate probability (small, multiple defects); or a normal result (no perfusion defect seen). Although, as in non-pregnant subjects, a negative result does not entirely exclude thrombosis, a normal result will often be considered as evidence of no PTE. If, however, there is continuing clinical suspicion, or when an intermediate result is obtained, spiral CT should be considered. It may lead to less radiation to the fetus than standard angiography by the femoral route, and even

V/Q scanning, but results in a substantial dose to the maternal breasts of around 2–3rads. In addition, although spiral CT has a high utility for central thrombosis, it may not reliably detect small peripheral events and has no proven track record in pregnancy. If there is sufficient diagnostic doubt, pulmonary angiography may be required. In such cases the brachial route should be preferred, as this results in a substantial reduction in the potential radiation exposure to the fetus. Many of the known side effects attributed to pulmonary angiography predate the introduction of low-ionic, low-osmolar contrast medium. Furthermore, pregnant women are less likely to have major cardiac, respiratory or renal disease, and are probably less susceptible to such side effects.

Risk assessment of VTE in pregnancy

In determining those at risk of VTE in pregnancy, many of the general risk factors in the population have limited utility. As noted above, this is due to the general absence of co-morbid conditions in this population. A number of factors increase the risk beyond that of pregnancy itself (Table 6.6), which includes: age, with those over 35 years at higher risk than those below (antenatal risk 0.06 versus 0.12% and postnatal risk 0.03 versus 0.07%); a family history of thrombosis; a past history of thrombosis; high parity (>3); operative delivery; other operative procedures; infection; nephrotic syndrome; pre-eclampsia;

Table 6.6 – Assessment of risks for venous thromboembolism (VTE) in pregnancy

Pre-existing	Family history VTE
	Past medical history VTE
	Thrombophilia
	Parity >3
	Obesity (>80kg or >25kg/m^2)
	Paraplegia
	Intravenous drug abuse
	Sickle-cell disease
	Essential thrombocythemia
	Nephrotic syndrome
	Inflammatory bowel disease
Acquired	Ovarian hyperstimulation
	Operative delivery
	Other operative procedure
	Infection
	Pre-eclampsia
	Abruption/major blood loss
	Dehydration
	Long-distance travel

obesity (weight >80kg or body mass index (BMI) >25kg/m^2); dehydration; inflammatory bowel disease; paraplegia; abruption; IV drug abuse; long-distance travel; and ovarian hyperstimulation in assisted conception.

As noted above, for those with a previous VTE, one prospective follow-up suggests that the risk of antepartum recurrence relates, predominantly, to those who have a detectable thrombophilia and/or a previous idiopathic VTE (recurrence rate around 6%). Whereas, those who have no thrombophilia, and where the previous VTE occurred in association with a temporary risk factor, appear to be at a very modest increased risk of antepartum recurrence.

A number of scenarios may present to the attending clinician. These include pregnant women with:

■ A family history of VTE in a first-degree relative (+/– known thrombophilia), but no personal history;

■ A family history of thrombophilia only;

■ A personal history of thrombophilia with no personal history of VTE (an incidental finding);

■ Previous VTE +/– known thrombophilia.

The risks associated with asymptomatic heritable thrombophilia are difficult to estimate with confidence from current studies, and any patient requires due consideration of the above categories. However, a rough guide of the risks associated with thrombophilia found in someone with no previous VTE or strong family history is shown (Table 6.7).

In general, those women with a history of VTE should undergo screening for thrombophilia. This should, if possible, be carried out before pregnancy, to allow detailed discussion and planning, as well as to avoid the difficulties in assessment of labile clotting factors in pregnancy (see Chapter 1).

Table 6.7 – Rough guide to thrombophilia and venous thromboembolism (VTE) risk related to pregnancy

Defect	Risk of VTE in pregnancy*
FV Leiden heterozygote	1 in 400
FV Leiden heterozygote + family history	1 in 100–200
FV Leiden homozygote	5 in 100
PT 20210A heterozygote	1 in 300
FV Leiden + PT 20210A compound heterozygote	4–5 in 100
Protein S deficiency	1 in 1000
Protein C deficiency	1 in 100
Antithrombin deficiency (mild – severe)	2–7 in 100

*Assumes 1 VTE in 1500 deliveries and an unselected population. AT, Antithrombin; F, Factor; PT, Prothrombin.

Prophylaxis of VTE in pregnancy

All pregnancies should be managed to minimize the risk of VTE (see Table 6.8), and prophylaxis with LMWH should be offered when appropriate (see Tables 6.9 and 6.10). All women with a previous VTE or thrombophilia should be encouraged to wear Class II graduated below-knee stockings (18–21mmHg at the ankle) for the whole of pregnancy and the puerperium. There is no evidence, however, that there is benefit in serial ultrasound screening of at-risk individuals, as DVT could occur between scans and, in pregnancy, serial ultrasound is likely to have <10% positive predictive value for DVT.

When antenatal prophylaxis is used, it should be commenced as soon as is practical after pregnancy is confirmed. Simlarly, postpartum prophylaxis should be commenced as soon as practical after delivery; however, if there has been a postpartum hemorrhage, therapy should be delayed. In circumstances of high thrombosis and hemorrhagic risk, there may be a place for intravenous UFH, as it has a shorter half-life and is more easily, and predictably, reversed with protamine sulfate.

If there has been regional analgesia, LMWH should be withheld until 4 hours have elapsed from the insertion, or removal, of the epidural catheter. In addition, placement of an epidural catheter should be carried out at least 12 hours after a prophylactic dose of LMWH and at least 24 hours after a therapeutic dose. Furthermore, catheter removal should also be delayed until 12 hours after the last LMWH dose.

Table 6.8 – Reduction of post-partum venous thromboembolism (VTE) risk

Monitor for clinical signs of VTE in the first week of the puerperium
Early mobilization and hydration
2+ risk factors: Compression stockings
3+ risk factors: LMWH/UFH for 3–5 days

LMWH, Low-molecular-weight heparin; UFH, Unfractionated heparin.

Table 6.9 – Low-molecular-weight heparin (LWMH) dosing*

	Standard prophylaxis (24 hourly)	High prophylaxis (12 hourly)	Treatment (12 hourly)
Tinzaparin	4500U	4500U	90U/kg
Dalteparin	5000U	5000U	90U/kg
Enoxaparin	40mg	40mg	1mg/kg

*Assumes normal body weight.

Table 6.10 – Low-molecular-weight heparin (LMWH) prophylaxis against venous thromboembolism (VTE) in pregnancy

Scenario	Antenatal LMWH	Postnatal LMWH	Dose	Comment
PMH VTE **On LT anticoagulant**	Yes	Yes	Treatment/high prophylactic	≤6 weeks PN
PMH VTE **No thrombophilia**	Yes If: previous • >1 VTE • Estrogen-linked VTE • Strong FH • Idopathic/persisting risk factor • Unusual VTE	Yes	Prophylactic	≤6 weeks PN
PMH VTE **+ thrombophilia** **(incl APAS)**	Yes	Yes	Prophylactic/ high prophylactic for AT deficiency	≤6 weeks PN
Thrombophilia, **no VTE** **excluding AT deficient** **or homozygote/** **combined heterozygote**	No	Yes	Prophylactic	≤6 weeks PN Especially if other risk factors
Thrombophilia, **no VTE** **AT deficient or** **homozygote/** **combined heterozygote**	Yes	Yes	Prophylactic	≤6 weeks PN
APA only **No previous VTE** **or recurrent** **loss**	No	No/Yes	Prophylactic	3–5 days PN if other risk factors
Multiple other **risk factors**	?	Yes	Prophylactic	3–5 days PN +/– AN

AN, Antenatal; APA, Antiphospholipid antibody; APAS, Antiphospholipid syndrome; AT, Antithrombin; FH, Family history; LT, Long term; PMH, Past medical history; PN, Postnatal

For those on treatment or high prophylactic doses of heparin, the dose should be reduced to a standard prophylactic dose the day before a planned delivery and continued throughout delivery at this dose. If the woman presents in labor, the treatment dose should be withheld and protamine sulfate used if required.

For those on prophylactic therapy, this can be withheld on the morning of an elective Cesarean section and given 3–4 hours (depending on the time elapsed from any LMWH injection) postoperatively. Each subject being considered for Cesarean section should undergo a risk assessment for VTE. Graduated below-knee stockings should be used and the presence of additional risk factors, such as obesity, an emergency Cesarian section during labor, older age (>35 years) and the presence of thrombophilia, should be considered when deciding if, in addition, heparin prophylaxis is indicated. Indeed, if there are three or more risk factors present, heparin prophylaxis should be considered for a vaginal delivery (see Table 6.8).

Travel and thrombosis

An association between immobilization and VTE was first reported in 1940, and a link with travel was reported in 1954. Although commonly associated with air travel, the risk appears to relate to any form of travel. It is becoming increasingly apparent that the risk is limited to journeys that are longer than 4 hours, and particularly those >8–11 hours. Overall, the increased risk is modest and is likely to be of the order of 2-fold, with <5% of all symptomatic VTE associated with travel. The majority of travel VTE is likely to present within 3 days of travel, although there may be an association of up to 1 month thereafter. In addition to lower limb immobility and stasis, a number of risk factors peculiar to air travel have been postulated. These include hypobaric hypoxia and low humidity (although there is likely to be <100ml of water loss in a long haul flight). However, such risks could be compounded by excess alcohol or dehydration. Overall, the risk of travel thrombosis appears to be most important in those with pre-existing risk factors for VTE. This includes those with a history of previous VTE, malignancy (within 2 years), a family history of VTE, a history of CIAO and those who have had recent (<3 months) total hip or knee replacement surgery. In addition, other factors, such as obesity, venous stasis and estrogen usage and, of course, pregnancy, should be considered. In small studies of selected populations, between 20 and 30% of subjects with a symptomatic DVT were observed to carry a mutation such as FV Leiden. The contribution of this mutation to travel VTE in those with no other risk factors requires further assessment.

To reduce the risk in pregnant travelers, there are a number of conservative measures that may be appropriate (Table 6.11). For flights >3–4 hours, the mother should be advised to carry out leg exercises, to request an aisle seat (as the majority of VTE related to air travel are seen in subjects sitting in window or middle seats), to walk around the cabin whenever possible, and to avoid dehyrdation or excess alcohol or caffeine. Pregnant women should also be advised to inform their insurance companies of the potential risk.

A small number of studies of non-pregnant subjects using graduated elastic stockings (predominantly 18–21mmHg at the ankle) have shown a reduction in the occurrence of Doppler-detected DVT related to long haul flights. Although

Table 6.11 – Reduction of travel venous thromboembolism (VTE) in pregnancy

Minimize alcohol/caffeine consumption
Avoid dehydration
Regular walks around the cabin and regular stops in car journeys
Isometric leg exercises
Class I to Class II graduated elastic stockings
Consider risk:benefit ratio of aspirin or low-molecular-weight heparin

there is no direct evidence in pregnancy, pregnant women with additional risk factors should wear such compression hosiery for flights >3–4 hours and, indeed, such stockings may be useful for prophylaxis, as well as comfort, in all pregnant women. For those with additional risk factors, chemical prophylaxis should also be considered and, where required, this should be achieved with LMWH. In such subjects a dose of, for example, 20–40mg of enoxaparin (or equivalent other LMWH), given 2–4 hours before each flight, would be appropriate.

Although there is reasonable evidence that aspirin may prevent VTE in the context of orthopedic surgery, there is no evidence, at present, that it will prevent travel-associated VTE. One study of long-haul flights has shown a neutral effect, with 13% of individuals reporting gastrointestinal (GI) side effects. Another has reported that around 50% of DVT associated with flights (>10 hours) occurred despite aspirin prophylaxis.

VTE treatment in pregnancy

At present there is little direct evidence to inform the management of acute VTE in pregnancy, with most information derived from non-pregnant cases. Confirmed VTE in pregnancy requires immediate therapy with intravenous, treatment-dose, UFH to achieve an APTT of at least 1.5 times the control value. It is recognized that, in non-pregnant subjects, treatment-dose LMWH is as effective as UFH, and this is increasingly used as the primary treatment of VTE; this use is now extending to pregnant subjects. However, given its shorter half-life and more complete reversibility with protamine, UFH is more appropriate if a VTE occurs within 2 weeks of the due delivery date. When UFH is used, it should be started with a 5000IU intravenous bolus, followed by 1000–2000IU/hour, commencing with 1000IU/hour. The APTT or anti-Xa assay should be assessed at around 6 hours after the bolus and, if a therapeutic dose is required, an APTT between 1.5 and 2.5, or an anti-Xa of 0.3–0.7IU/ml, should be achieved within the first 24 hours of therapy.

If LMWH is used as primary treatment, monitoring of the anti-Xa level is of value, given the changes in LMWH kinetics with increasing gestation. A target of 0.5–1.2 anti-Xa units is desirable at 3–6 hours after dosing, but dosing requires due consideration of the relative IIa/Xa activity of an individual LMWH.

Treatment should be continued for 3–6 months after the event and should include the puerperium in all cases. Whether treatment should be continued for 6 or 12 weeks after delivery is not clear, but may depend on whether the VTE occurred early or late in pregnancy. In any case, it is sensible to review all patients at 3 months to determine if there are persisting risk factors. Whether it is safe to reduce the dose of heparin after the first 2–3 weeks of therapy is also not clear, but a change to LMWH with, or without, a dose reduction is widely practiced, especially if there is a high risk of osteoporosis or hemorrhage. In all cases, the platelet count should be measured at least after 7 days of therapy, and perhaps more frequently if there is to be prolonged use of UFH. In those with an antenatal VTE, an individual decision is required as to whether heparin or warfarin should be used for continuing treatment in the puerperium.

Vena cava filters

There is limited experience of vena cava filters in the management of pregnancy-related VTE. However, as in the non-pregnant, the general indications are: emboli that recur despite adequate anticoagulation; a significant contraindication to full-dose anticoagulation after a VTE; or marked patient debility, where it is perceived that a further embolic event may be fatal. The value and safety of a filter to permit a reduction in the dose of heparin when VTE occurs close to delivery, and the need for a filter solely on the basis of a VTE in someone with patent foramen ovale, both require further study.

Although early filters carried a significant risk of caval thrombosis (around 85%) and persisting lower limb venous insufficiency, more recent devices are conical in shape: this allows formed clot to be concentrated at the apex of the device and permits continued flow across the filter, which should lead to physiological lysis of any formed clot. Such newer devices have been reported to have a long-term patency rate of 95% and a risk of recurrence of PTE of <4%. However, the lifelong placement of such filters has been associated with a number of complications, including: device failure; device migration into the right atrium; penetration through the vessel wall; an increased risk of pelvic or leg thrombosis and; the possibility of small emboli occurring through small or collateral vessels.

From the limited experience of newer devices in pregnancy, they are associated with a favorable maternal and fetal outcome, although, around 25% of subjects may have evidence of persisting lower limb edema well after delivery. More recently, there have been a number of case reports of retrievable filters being used when VTE occurs at, or near, delivery. The overall role and safety of this modality of therapy in pregnancy is not yet clear.

Thrombolytic therapy and embolectomy

In those patients with PTE accompanied by cardiac compromise (or perhaps PTE with right ventricular dysfunction alone), treatment with thrombolytic therapy, or embolectomy, should be considered.

Thrombolysis has been achieved with streptokinase and recombinant tPA (rtPA) in pregnancy. Both of these activate plasminogen to plasmin, which cleaves fibrin (as well as fibrinogen, FVIII and FV).

As noted in Chapter 1, tPA preferentially activates plasminogen in the presence of fibrin and this should result in a more local lytic action. rtPA does not cross the placenta and is not antigenic. Streptokinase does cross the placenta, but not to a degree that results in lysis in the developing fetus. However, streptokinase is antigenic and at least 6 months should elapse between doses. One further lytic agent is urokinase (see Chapter 1), which does cross the placenta, but it is not clear whether this causes a significant problem in the fetus.

From the limited case-report evidence of thrombolysis in pregnancy (employed for a variety of indications), a maternal hemorrhage rate of between 1 and 8% is to be expected. There is low maternal mortality (<1%), which is broadly comparable with that in the non-pregnant. However, the use of any such therapy is associated with a 2–6% fetal loss rate and a comparable risk of premature delivery. Such data must be interpreted with caution, however, as they may be influenced by the severity of the indication for such therapy. From the limited reports, there is no clear evidence of superiority of any one particular agent in the management of VTE.

One further advance is the use of catheter-directed thrombolysis. This requires expertise in pulmonary artery catheterization and there is a need for maternal radiation exposure to permit catheter placement. However, at present, there is insufficient evidence to suggest that this approach is superior to standard therapy in the management of either DVT or PTE in pregnancy.

There is very little information on the use of embolectomy in pregnancy. Its use has been limited to severe maternal disease and is associated with a significant fetal loss rate of 20–40%, related to the need for cardiac bypass. However, this may be of secondary importance given the severity of the maternal illness.

References

Chan et al. 2000. Anticoagulation of pregnant women with mechanical heart valves: a systematic review of the literature. Arch Int Med, 160, 191–6.

CHAPTER 7
Thrombophilia and pregnancy outcome

Serious pregnancy complications, including pre-eclampsia (PET), fetal loss, intrauterine growth restriction (IUGR) and placental abruption, occur in up to 5% of women of reproductive age, and may be related to alterations in placental perfusion and development. In the past few years maternal carriage of a number of heritable thrombophilias, or thrombophilias with a mixture of heritable and environmental influences, have been linked with such pregnancy complications. Although a link between the thrombophilias and pregnancy-associated venous thromboembolism (VTE: Table 7.1) is consistent with their potential to generate an excess of thrombin and fibrin. The mechanism for their role in other

Table 7.1 – Relative risk of venous thromboembolism (VTE)

Event	Relative risk
Pregnancy	4
Puerperium	14
Cancer	10
Medical immobilization	11
Postoperative	6–10
COCP	4–6
HRT	2–4
↑ FVIIIC	4–6
↑ HCY	2–4
PC/PS/AT deficiency	Around 10
Family history	Around 10
Heterozygous FV Leiden	5–8
Homozygous FV Leiden	50–80
Heterozygous PT 202010A	2–4
Homozygous PT 202010A	10
Antitphospholipid syndrome	7–9

AT, Antithrombin; COCP, Combined oral contraceptive pill; F, Factor; HCY, Homocysteine; HRT, Hormone replacement therapy; PC, Protein C; PS, Protein S; PT, Prothrombin.

pregnancy disorders is not so obvious, but could also be linked with alterations in both thrombin generation and endothelial function.

As detailed in Chapter 1, thrombin is the pivotal protein in the coagulation process. In addition to a wide variety of pro-coagulant functions (including platelet activation, conversion of fibrinogen to fibrin and activation of Factors (F) Vc and VIIIc), it also has an anticoagulant function via thrombomodulin and the generation of activated protein C (aPC). Thus, via this negative feedback, thrombin ultimately regulates its own generation. Adequate anticoagulant functioning of thrombin via aPC depends upon intact functioning of the endothelium, adequate levels of the components of the protein C/protein S system and a normal sensitivity to the effects of aPC. Thrombin also participates directly in tissue remodeling, wound repair, leukocyte chemotaxis, leukocyte adhesion, vascular contraction and vascular permeability, via interactions with specific endothelial and leukocyte thrombin receptors.

Although endothelial activation is a feature of normal pregnancy, heightened activation has been linked with disorders such as PET. Any condition, such as a thrombophilia, that has the potential to increase thrombin generation, or alter endothelial function, may be capable, therefore, of influencing placental function and thereby fetal development. Maternal thrombophilia may, by excessive thrombin generation, also alter the maternal response to the feto-placental unit. This may, for example, contribute to the maternal presentation of PET. Whether fetal inheritance of paternal thrombophilia contributes to these conditions has not been fully examined, but could also be important in the generation of these fetal and maternal disorders.

Heritable thrombophilias

Protein S deficiency

Protein S is a vitamin K-dependent, single-chain glycoprotein, which is synthesized in the liver and vascular endothelium, and acts mainly as a cofactor to aPC in the inactivation of FVIIIa and FVa (Figure 7.1). The plasma level of protein S depends upon age, sex, lipid levels, estrogen, oral anticoagulant usage and the presence of acute thrombosis (Table 7.2). In the plasma, around 60% of circulating protein S is bound to C4b binding protein, and only free protein S can function as a cofactor to aPC. The binding protein itself may also function as a link between thrombosis and complement activation. Indeed, as C4b increases in pregnancy, the binding protein also contributes to the physiological reduction in protein S levels seen with increasing gestation.

Heritable protein S deficiency is transmitted as an autosomal dominant trait. Those with heterozygous deficiency are at increased risk of VTE, as well as warfarin-induced skin necrosis. Homozygote deficiency is extremely rare, as it is usually associated with neonatal purpura fulminans and fetal or perinatal death. However, there are reports of homozygous individuals who have survived long enough until life-long anticoagulation can be established. Although there is no agreed classification of inherited protein S deficiency, three subclasses have been proposed. These result from mutations which lead to either:

■ A reduction in total and free protein S antigen levels;
■ A reduction in free protein S antigen and activity, without a reduction in the total protein S level;
■ A reduction in protein S activity only, without a reduction in antigen.

However, as some functional protein S assays give falsely low protein S activity assessments when FV Leiden is present, there is no universally accepted (or practical) definition of functional protein S deficiency.

With allowance for this, the prevalence of heterozygous protein S deficiency in the general population is of the order of 1 in 300–400. Heterozygous deficiency carries around a 10-fold risk of VTE, but is found in <5% of those with a history of venous thrombosis. At present, however, there is no substantive evidence which links protein S deficiency and arterial thrombosis in adults. As there are a number of mutations which can result in protein S deficiency, the diagnosis (unless a specific mutation is known in other family members) is made by assessment of plasma protein S levels (Table 7.2).

Protein C deficiency

Like protein S, protein C is also a vitamin K-dependent glycoprotein. It is synthesized in the liver and, when activated, inactivates FVa and FVIIIa in the presence of protein S. Its plasma levels are influenced by age, sex, lipid levels, and the presence of liver disease, renal disease, acute thrombosis, disseminated intravascular coagulation (DIC) or warfarin use. Higher levels can be seen in the puerperium and in subjects on oral contraceptives (see Table 7.2).

As with protein S, heritable deficiency is transmitted as an autosomal trait and heterozygous deficiency increases the risk of thrombosis around 10-fold. The

Figure 7.1 Thrombophilia

The principal points of the coagulation cascade that are associated with thrombophilia are shown. The actions of antithrombin (AT – previously called antithrombin III), which are reduced by AT deficiency are shown. Protein C (PC), via activated protein C (aPC) and its cofactor protein S (PS), acts to inactivate Factor (F) Va (Va) and FVIIIa (VIIIa). The action on FVa is impaired when there is the FV Leiden (FVL) mutation, and the action on FVIIIa is impaired when there is an elevation of FVIIIc. This occurs in pregnancy, during the acute phase reaction and also in association with the combined oral contraceptive or hormone replacement therapy. Elevated FIXc levels are also an independent risk factor for venous thromboembolism (VTE). Elevated fibrinogen levels and antibodies to phospholipid are associated with an increased risk of VTE and arterial thrombosis. Ca²⁺, Calcium; Plipid, phospholipid; PTG20210A, prothrombin G20210A mutation; TAT, thrombin–antithrombin complex; TF, tissue factor.

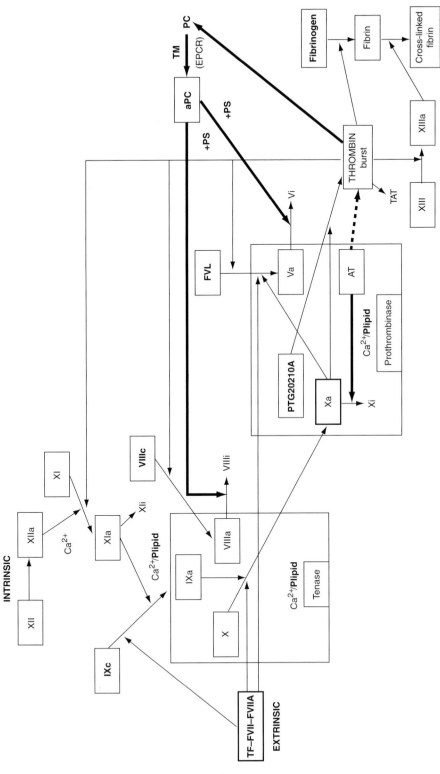

Table 7.2 – Factors influencing plasma thrombophilia assessments

Thrombophilia	Factor	Effect
Hyperhomocysteine (hyperHCY)	Sample anticoagulant	Different HCY levels with different anticoagulants (citrate or EDTA) or anticoagulant concentrations
	Time to plasma separation	Separate plasma <1 hour to avoid higher HCY from ongoing wbc metabolism
	Fasting versus non-fasting	Role not defined in predicting risk
	Methionine loading versus no methionine loading	Role not defined in predicting risk
	Pregnancy	Reduces HCY level
	Renal impairment	Increases HCY level
	Hypothyroidism	Increases HCY level
	Haematinic deficiency	Increases HCY level
	Contraceptives	Reduces HCY level
Protein C (PC) activity	Acute thrombosis	Reduces PC level
	Coumarins	Reduces PC level
	Pregnancy	No gestation effect but non-pregnant ranges may not be appropriate Levels may increase in early puerperium
	Hyperlipidemia	Increases PC level
Protein S (PS) antigen	Acute thrombosis	Reduces PS level
	Coumarins	Reduces PS level
	Pregnancy	Reduces PS level
AT activity	Acute thrombosis	Reduces AT level
	Pregnancy	No gestation effect but non-pregnant ranges may not be appropriate
	Heparin	Reduces AT level
Lupus inhibitor	Anticoagulants	Unreliable result (?except low-molecular-weight heparin)
aPCR (APTT-based)	Anticoagulants	Unreliable result
	Blood group non-O	Increases aPCR
	Pregnancy	Increases aPCR
	Oral contraceptives	Increases aPCR
	Hormone replacement therapy	Increases aPCR
	Body mass index	Increases aPCR
	Blood pressure	Increases aPCR
aPCR (thrombin-generation)	Anticoagulants	Unreliable result
	Oral contraceptives	Increases aPCR
Factor (F) VIIIc	Blood group non-O	Increases FVIIIc
	Pregnancy	Increases FVIIIc
	Contraceptives	Increases FVIIIc
	Acute phase response	Increases FVIIIc
	Warfarin	No effect

homozygous state is also associated with neonatal purpura fulminans. In such circumstances the use of human-derived protein C concentrate may rescue such individuals until lifelong anticoagulation can be established. Heterozygous deficiency has been estimated to occur in 1 in 300–500 of the population, but is also found in <5% of those with venous thrombosis. As with protein S, there is no evidence that protein C deficiency is linked with arterial thrombosis in adults. In studies investigating blood donor populations, the majority of individuals identified (either biochemically or genetically) are symptom free. Protein C deficiency has been classified into two types:

- Type 1: a quantitative reduction in functionally normal protein C;
- Type 2: a level of protein C activity that is less than the antigen level; a deficiency that results from the production of a functionally abnormal protein C molecule.

These deficiencies can result from a number of genetic mutations and, as a result, the diagnosis of protein C deficiency is made from the detection of reduced plasma levels, unless there is a known mutation in other family members (see Table 7.2).

Antithrombin deficiency

Although originally termed antithrombin III, the use of III is now considered redundant. This glycoprotein is capable of inactivating most of the activated clotting factors (including FVIIa bound to tissue factor (TF)). The presence of heparin increases its ability to inactivate FXa and FIIa (thrombin) around 1000-fold. Functional plasma levels are reduced in acute thrombosis, DIC, and in patients receiving heparin therapy. Otherwise, there is little variation in plasma levels with age and sex, and levels often remain within the non-pregnant range during pregnancy.

Antithrombin deficiency is inherited as an autosomal trait, which, in its severe heterozygous form, increases the risk of VTE around 20-fold and in its less severe form around 10-fold. A homozygous severe deficiency is probably incompatible with survival, but milder homozygous deficiencies may be amenable to replacement with human-derived or recombinant antithrombin concentrate until lifelong anticoagulation can be established. A number of genetic mutations, which alter either the clotting or heparin binding sites, are described. More severe defects reduce antigen and activity equally, and lesser defects result in less activity than antigen. Akin to the situation with protein C and S, the number of potential mutations means that deficiency is routinely diagnosed on the basis of reduced plasma levels. Again, in some instances, it may be possible to detect, or exclude, a mutation that is known to have occurred in other family members. The prevalence of defects in the general population leading to a severe deficiency is of the order of 1 in 4000–5000, although milder defects are more common and may be as prevalent as 1 in 400. As with protein C and S deficiency, antithrombin is found infrequently in those with VTE (<3%), but is more often associated with more severe disease, or disease onset at an early age. Indeed, around 50% of severe heterozygotes experience thrombosis before the age of 30 years. Akin to the situation with protein S and protein C, there is no evidence that antithrombin deficiency is associated with arterial thrombosis.

FV Leiden

FV Leiden occurs as a result of a G→A mutation at position 1691 in the gene coding for coagulation FV. It is the commonest heritable cause of resistance to aPC (see below) and results in a change in one of the parts of the FV molecule that is the target for cleavage by aPC. It is inherited as an autosomal dominant condition with both heterozygotes and homozygotes surviving into adulthood. Heterozygotes are reasonably common in European populations, with a prevalence of between 2 and 15%, but are less common, or even absent, in other populations. In those of European extraction, FV Leiden is found in its homozygous form in around 1 in 1000. Heterozygotes are also found in around 50% of those with a history of VTE. In heterozygotes it carries around a 5-8-fold risk of VTE, with a higher risk (around 50–80-fold) in homozygotes, and an increasing risk associated with increasing age (Table 7.3). Given its high prevalence, it is not unusual to find it in combination with other thrombophilic disorders. Whether, in combination with smoking, it has a causal role in myocardial infarction is a matter of topical debate, but there is no evidence linking FV Leiden with arterial thrombosis in any other circumstances. Other heritable causes of aPC resistance

Table 7.3 – Age and absolute venous thromboembolism (VTE) risk

Age	Subgroups	VTE risk
Child	All	1/million/year
<45 years	All	1/10000/year
	♀ heterozygous Factor (F) V Leiden	1/1500/year
	♀ on COCP	1/2500/year
	♀ heterozygous FV Leiden on COCP	1/350/year
45–75 years	All	1/1000/year
	Menopausal ♀	1/500/year
	on hormone replacement therapy (HRT)	
	Menopausal ♀ + heterozygous FV Leiden	1/150/year
	Menopausal ♀ + heterozygous FV Leiden on HRT	1/70/year
>75 years	All	1/100–400/year

COCP, Combined oral contraceptive pill

include two other point mutations in the FV gene (FV Cambridge and FV Hong Kong) and a group of FV polymorphisms, known as the HR2 haplotype. At present, the clinical impact of these alterations is unknown.

Prothrombin G20210A mutation

A mutation in the gene coding for the prothrombin molecule was described in 1996 (Poort SR, *et al*, 1996). This results from a single base substitution (G→A) at position 20210, which leads, by an as yet unknown mechanism, to higher levels of circulating prothrombin. It is found in 1–2% of Caucasians, but is more common in those of Mediterranean descent. It confers a 2–4- and around 10-fold risk of VTE in heterozygotes and homozygotes, respectively. There is also likely to be an even higher risk in those who are compound heterozygotes for the prothrombin G20210A and FV Leiden mutations. Like FV Leiden, any potential link between the mutation, smoking and myocardial infarction in young women is not yet resolved, and there is no link with arterial thrombosis in other circumstances.

Thermolabile methylene tetrahydrofolate reductase (MTHFR C677T)

As noted in Chapter 3, the manufacture of DNA results in the generation of homocysteine (HCY). The blood level of HCY is under the influence of the enzymes and hematinic cofactors of the HCY – methionine pathway. One of the enzymes of this pathway is methylene tetrahydrofolate reductase (MTHFR), and a specific–point mutation in its gene results in relative thermolability of the enzyme called MTHFR C677T. This mutation occurs in the homozygous form in 5–15% and in its heterozygous form in up to 35% of Caucasians. At present, there is insufficient evidence to suggest that this mutation has a role, independent from HCY, on the occurrence of venous or arterial thrombosis. For relationship to pregnancy complications see 'Hyperhomocysteinemia' (p. 135).

Dysfibrinogenemia

See Chapter 4.

Heritable thrombophilia and pre-eclampsia (PET)

PET is a multisystem disorder that is characterized by hypertension, renal dysfunction and fluid retention during pregnancy in someone who has no pre-existing hypertension or renal dysfunction. It is defined as the development of hypertension (defined as a blood pressure of ≥140/90mmHg, or a blood pressure that is ≥30/15mmHg over the subject's baseline level on at least two occasions, 6 hours apart) accompanied by the development of proteinuria (defined as >300mg/24 hours, or 30mg/dl on a confirmed random sample), indicating renal damage. Formal quantification of the level of proteinuria is most often assessed by obtaining a 24-hour collection. In practice, however, the diagnosis of significant proteinuria is often accepted as the presence of >2+ proteinuria on repeated urinary dipstick testing. Once established, PET progresses at a variable and unpredictable pace until delivery. Both the hypertension and the proteinuria resolve postnatally.

Although hypertension without proteinuria (i.e. pregnancy-induced hypertension) can lead to significant disease, it carries a much better prognosis for the mother and the fetus than PET. At the other extreme, around one third of subjects with PET present with seizures. This, termed eclampsia, can be complicated by coma, neurological deficit and, in a small percentage, with intracerebral hemorrhage. It is due to cerebral involvement of the disease and is thought to involve vasospasm leading to ischemia, disruption of the blood–brain barrier and cerebral edema. Forty-four per cent of cases of eclampsia occur postnatally, 38% in the antepartum period and 18% intrapartum.

Hemolysis, elevated liver enzymes, (HELLP) syndrome and low platelets is a serious manifestation occurring in 4–12% of women with PET. Hemolysis reflects microangiopathic hemolytic anemia (MAHA) and the elevated transaminases reflect liver dysfunction occuring through vascular damage. Thrombocytopenia reflects a coagulation disturbance, although in HELLP syndrome the main coagulation parameters (activated partial thromboplastin time (APTT), prothrombin time (PT) and thrombin clotting time (TT) remain within normal limits. Since elevated blood pressure is not always present at the onset of this condition, it may be confused with other conditions causing thrombocytopenia or abnormal liver function tests. HELLP syndrome is more likely to occur in multiparous women. The infants of HELLP syndrome mothers also have an increased risk of thrombocytopenia, although this most likely results from a combination of fetal stress and ineffective platelet development.

The presence of hyperuricemia can be useful diagnostically, as it can help distinguish between these pregnancy-induced hypertensive disorders and pre-existing hypertension. An elevated plasma uric acid level also occurs before the onset of proteinuria and is a useful marker of disease severity, since it increases with disease progression. The normal range for serum uric acid levels is, however, lower during pregnancy than in non-pregnant women. Hence, at 32 weeks' gestation, the upper limit of normal is 0.34 μmol/l and at 36 weeks gestation is 0.39μmol/l. Raised serum uric acid levels during pregnancy are best regarded as an indicator of impaired renal function and renal blood flow. In women with PET, a rising plasma urea or creatinine indicates a worsening of the disease. A low platelet count occurs in normal pregnancy (see Chapter 8) and a falling platelet count is seen in PET, but this is an inconsistent feature of the disease.

PET remains a poorly understood disorder that complicates around 3% of pregnancies. A number of maternal constitutional risk factors have been described (Table 7.4). In addition, a multiple pregnancy, maternal age (<20 or >35 years), a history of previous PET, a maternal family history of PET, the presence of diabetes mellitus, migraine, as well as some fetal factors, such as hydrops fetalis, hydatidiform mole, triploidy and trisomy 13, are also linked with a higher risk of PET. In recent years a link with various inherited and/or acquired thrombophilias has been made (see Table 7.4). The etiology of the condition remains unknown, but is generally accepted to be related to abnormal placentation, and probably represents a failure of the normal immune tolerance that the mother should have to the presence of the fetus.

In addition to the similarities between the placental pathology of PET (acute atheroma – a necrotizing arteriopathy with fibrinoid necrosis and lipid-laden macrophage accumulation in the placental bed) and cardiovascular pathology, PET is accompanied by acute changes in coagulation, including a supraphysiological increase in von Willebrand's Factor (vWF), FVIIIc and TF expression, as well as platelet activation and a reduction in antithrombin activity. These changes can progress to encompass the syndrome of disseminated intravascular coagulation. PET also carries an increased risk of IUGR, and women with a past history of PET appear more likely to have higher circulating levels of coagulation factors, lipids and insulin resistance. This may be reflected in a higher risk of cardiovascular disease in later life for the mother, as well as a higher risk of vascular

Table 7.4 – Pre-eclampsia (PET) risk

	Risk factor	Relative risk
Thrombophilia	AT/protein C (PC) deficiency	?
	Factor (F) V Leiden	2–5*
	Hyperhomocysteine	5†
	MTHFR C677T	2*
	Protein S	10*
	APA	4*
	Prothrombin G20210A	2–7*
	Acquired activated PC resistance	7†
Constitutional	PMH chronic HBP	10
	Primigravida/primipaternity	5
	Body mass index (BMI)/waist circumference	2.2–2.7‡
	PMH pre-eclampsia	8
	Smoking	0.5

*The risks associated with individual thrombophilias relate predominantly to retrospective studies, and in many cases these have not been confirmed in all studies and particularly in prospective series.
†The relative risk relates to the risk in the highest quartile compared with the lowest.
‡The relative risk of PET with a waist circumference (at pregnancy presentation) of 80cm compared with a waist circumference of <80cm, or of a BMI >26kg/m² (at pregnancy presentation) when compared with a BMI <26kg/m².
APA, Antiphospholipid; AT, Antithrombin; HBP, High blood pressure; PMH, Past medical history

disease and Type 2 diabetes mellitus in later life in those infants with a history of IUGR.

A link between a history of previous VTE and the risk of PET has been reported in one study, and several case-control studies have found at least one inherited thrombophilia in anything up to 70% of women with PET (when compared with <20% in control subjects). A number of studies have specifically examined aPC resistance (both FV Leiden and acquired) and the risk of PET. In those studies reporting a positive link, the magnitude of the risk attributed to heterozygous FV Leiden is between 2- and 5-fold. In some of these studies it has also been suggested that thrombophilia may be associated with more severe PET. In the main, however, a positive link between thrombophilia has only been seen in retrospective studies, and prospective studies have not confirmed any link. Consequently, further work is required to determine whether this disparity in evidence relates to differences in the prevalence of FV Leiden in the different populations, differences in the severity of PET in different studies, or to a more accurate diagnosis in prospective investigations.

The prothrombin G20210A mutation has also been linked to an increased risk of PET (between 2- and 7-fold) in a small number of studies, although the majority of reports have not found any association. Protein S deficiency has also been found in up to 25% of subjects with a history of PET. However, as there is a physiological fall in protein S in normal pregnancy, the exact contribution of abnormal levels to the development of PET requires further study. At present, due to the relative rarity of the disorders, there is insufficient evidence to give an estimate of risk for those with antithrombin (AT) or protein C deficiency. Although MTHFR C677T has also been linked with around 2-fold risk of PET in some reports, the majority of studies have not found an independent role for this genetic variant. These studies suggest that levels of the hematinic cofactors of the HCY–methionine pathway (such as folic acid) may be considerably more important than the C677T in the causation of disease.

Although this potential involvement of heritable thrombophilia in the causation of PET is intriguing, and may shed light on the pathogenesis of this disease, there is no evidence that identification of thrombophilia carriers would reliably identify those at risk of developing PET. Furthermore, there is no substantial evidence that reduction of thrombin generation in such individuals, by the use of anticoagulants, would result in a beneficial pregnancy outcome. At present, then, there is no case that routine, or even selected, thrombophilia screening of individuals (based upon past medical or obstetric history) would be of benefit in the management of this condition.

Heritable thrombophilia and intrauterine growth restriction (IUGR)

A few studies have specifically addressed the impact of heritable thrombophilia on IUGR. In some studies, carriage of a thrombophilia has been associated with at least a 2-fold risk of IUGR (most commonly defined as growth to less than the

10th centile), with a relative 4–7-fold risk for carriage of either FV Leiden or pro-thrombin G20210A. However, as with other pregnancy complications, a number of studies have not shown any link between IUGR and heritable thrombophilia. Further work, perhaps concentrating on births of <5th centile, are required before a definite link with thrombophilia can be proven.

Heritable thrombophilia and fetal loss

Pregnancy loss occurs in 12–20% of first pregnancies, with two losses affecting around 5% of women, and three or more losses (recurrent pregnancy loss) affecting around 2% of women of reproductive age. It is likely that the majority of losses related to immune, karyotypic, endocrine or other fetal/maternal defects and are not directly related to thrombosis. However, the placenta in fetal loss may show evidence of infarction, thrombosis, and/or perivillous fibrin depo-sition. Indeed, these changes can be seen in fetal loss associated with throm-bophilia, but they are not always evident and are reasonably common even in the absence of any known thrombophilia.

On the basis of limited evidence protein C, protein S and AT deficiency have all been associated with around a 2-fold risk of recurrent pregnancy loss. Fetal loss also appears to be more common in those members of a thrombophilic family who have the deficiency when compared with those family members who do not. Although there is likely to be a link with fetal loss, because of the relative rarity of these deficiencies, the magnitude of the risk and whether the risk relates exclusively to late or early loss is not yet resolved.

In the majority of studies, a 2–7-fold increased risk of recurrent loss has been associated with carriage of the FV Leiden mutation, suggesting that FV Leiden is an independent risk factor for fetal loss. Overall, it appears that this risk is more likely to be related to pregnancy loss occurring after the first trimester (in particular after 24 weeks). The risk of loss is also likely to be higher in subjects who are homozygote for FV Leiden (perhaps two times greater than heterozy-gotes), or those who have a combination of defects (such as FV Leiden and antiphospholipid syndrome, where the risk may be as high as 14-fold). Despite this, the vast majority of subjects who are heterozygous for FV Leiden have a normal pregnancy outcome. This suggests that other factors, perhaps including fetal FV Leiden inheritance, may play a part in fetal loss associated with FV Leiden.

So far, the role of the prothrombin G20210A mutation in fetal loss has not yet been confirmed, although some studies suggest that it too may be associated with a 2–3-fold risk of all recurrent pregnancy losses, including both single late and recurrent early loss. This may be particularly so if the prothrombin G20210A mutation is combined with other defects.

It is unlikely that heterozygous carriage of the MTHFR C677T variant results in any increase in risk of pregnancy complications. Although a few studies have reported that homozygous carriage of the mutation increases the risk of placental abruption and recurrent pregnancy loss, the vast majority of studies and met-analyses have found that, despite a 3–4 increased risk of recurrent fetal loss associated with hyperhomocysteinemia (see below), there appears to be little independent contribution from the MTHFR C677T variant.

Thrombophilia with genetic and acquired components
Activated protein C resistance (aPCR)

Resistance to the anticoagulant effects of aPC (aPCR) was originally described in association with antiphospholipid antibodies. Subsequently, an examination of the effect of exogenously added aPC on the APTT of subjects with a personal or family history of VTE demonstrated that aPCR could be inherited. The addition of aPC (by inactivating FVa and FVIIIa in the sample) should lead to a prolongation of the APTT. In subjects with FV Leiden, addition of aPC does prolong the APTT (as FV Leiden produces a relative, not absolute, resistance to aPC), but to a much lesser degree than in those not carrying the mutation. Indeed, this forms the basis of an APTT-based assay to detect the presence of FV Leiden. This test is, however, also influenced by other factors. In particular, blood groups other than O (non-O), higher plasma FVIIIc levels, combined oral contraceptives, pregnancy, hormone replacement therapy, antiphospholipid antibodies and the presence of the prothrombin G20210A mutation all lead to greater aPCR when assessed by this test. The test is also unreliable in the presence of anticoagulants. To render the APTT test more specific for heritable mutations in the FV gene, the patient's plasma sample can be pre-diluted with FV-deficient plasma. This modification excludes these other influences, including anticoagulants, rendering it highly sensitive and specific for mutations in FV such as FV Leiden.

There are other methods for detecting aPCR. One method is an assay essentially based upon the PT rather than the APTT. In this test the PT is modified so that the end point is the amount of thrombin (not fibrin) generated with time. To detect FV Leiden, the amount of thrombin generated after the sample is activation by FVIIa/TF is assessed. The test is repeated with exogenously added aPC, and the difference in the amount of thrombin generated leads to an aPCR index. This test is particularly sensitive (more so than the APTT-based test) to the different levels of aPCR generated by the second and third generation oral contraceptive pills.

Both the unmodified APTT- and thrombin generation-based tests may be capable of giving more information than simply the detection of genetic defects such as FV Leiden, and the term 'acquired aPCR' has been coined for resistance which is found without FV Leiden (or other mutations in FV). Indeed, these tests may have, ultimately, a value in assessing overall arterial and venous thrombotic potential. However, further work is required to standardize these tests before they can become useful for the prediction of disease. Preliminary evidence does suggest, however, that higher aPCR is associated with an increased risk of both arterial and venous thrombosis.

aPCR and pregnancy outcome

As noted in Chapter 1, in around 80% of normal subjects, increasing gestation leads to increasing acquired aPCR (as detected by the APTT method). In pregnancy, higher levels of acquired aPCR correlate with higher FVIIIc and FVc, and lower protein S levels. In one study, those with the greatest resistance in early pregnancy had a 7-fold increased risk of PET developing later in that pregnancy. There may also be a link between the degree of acquired aPCR and fetal weight, although no relationship between aPCR (when assessed during pregnancy) and fetal loss has yet been described. However one study has reported that acquired aPCR (assessed after pregnancy) is more common in those with a history of PET or fetal loss. Although these observations are interesting, standardization of the assay techniques is required before any clinical use can be made of the APTT-based aPC resistance in the detection or prevention of disease.

At present there is also very little information on the relationship between acquired aPCR (assessed by thrombin generation) and pregnancy outcome, although preliminary results suggest that higher resistance in early pregnancy does not predict an increased risk of PET.

Hyperhomocysteinemia

Mild–moderate hyperhomocysteinemia (hyperHCY) is found in around 5% of North European populations, and may be twice as common in those with a history of VTE and 2–5 times more common in those with atherosclerotic disease. Although this is not a substantial risk, it is of interest, as hyperHCY may be amenable to treatment with folic acid. However, the evidence that such intervention reduces the risk of coronary artery disease is disputed and, at present, there is no evidence at all that folic acid will substantially reduce the risk of recurrence of VTE. As noted in Chapter 3, the level of HCY is dependent on several key enzymes in the HCY-methionine pathway, as well as the level of the vitamin cofactors of these reactions (vitamins B_{12}, vitamin B_6 and folic acid).

HyperHCY and pregnancy outcome

As detailed in Chapter 3, hyperHCY is associated with an increased risk of spina bifida and around a 2-fold risk has also been observed in homozygotes for the MTHFR C677T variant, with a similar size of risk observed with other polymorphisms in the HCY-methionine pathway. As the use of routine periconceptual folic acid reduces the risk of neural tube defects by around 50%, it would seem likely that the risk of neural tube defects depends not only on the presence of these polymorphisms but also on the mother's hematinic cofactor levels.

There is some evidence that links hyperHCY with, predominantly, early fetal loss. It is difficult to determine the exact magnitude of the risk as: studies used differing definitions of hyperHCY; in some, the subjects were receiving routine folic acid prophylaxis; and whilst some studies assessed HCY out-with pregnancy, others made the diagnosis during the affected pregnancy. The evidence that exists, however, suggests that the actual degree of risk may be directly correlated with the plasma HCY level, with higher levels leading to greater risk. In those studies showing a positive association, the risk of first loss varied from 3- to 7-fold, with the recurrent loss risk some 3–4-fold increased. Some studies have also shown a link between hyperHCY and later pregnancy loss, although this has not been seen in all positive studies.

In subjects with hyperHCY (diagnosed out-with pregnancy), there is also an increased risk of PET, with the highest risk seen in those with the highest levels of HCY. In particular, those with levels >9–11µmol/l are likely to have around a 5-fold higher risk of PET when compared with those with lower levels. The greatest risk is found in primigravid subjects, where the risk may be as high as 20-fold. In one study, which assessed HCY levels in early pregnancy, a link between the HCY level and the development of PET in the same pregnancy has also been reported, although this finding has not been confirmed.

At present there is no convincing evidence that folate supplementation will reduce the risk of recurrence of PET or the occurrence of fetal loss. However, as folic acid supplementation is routinely carried out in most developed countries, the main issue may be what is the appropriate and safe dose (400µg versus 5mg) and what the duration of such therapy should be, rather than to whether it should be prescribed or not. If HCY does influence pregnancy outcome, it would appear likely that alterations in fetal/placental DNA replication, as well as thrombosis, are involved.

Elevated FVIIIc, FIXc and fibrinogen levels

In non-pregnant subjects, plasma FVIIIc levels in excess of 150IU/dl are associated with a 5-fold increased risk of VTE, and elevated levels are found in around 25% of subjects at least 6 months after VTE. There is also an association between high FVIIIc levels and an increased risk of ischemic heart disease and cerebral ischemia of arterial origin. Elevated FVIIIc levels are found in around 10% of the general population and are more common in subjects of blood groups other than O (i.e. groups A and B, and perhaps particularly those with genotypes AA, AB or BB). This relation with blood group is consistent with over 40 years of data suggesting that blood groups have a bearing on the risk of both VTE and arterial thrombosis. The level of FVIIIc also relates to APTT-assessed aPCR (see above). However, an independent role for FVIIIc in pregnancy complications may be difficult to define, as pregnancy is associated with a marked physiological rise in FVIIIc with increasing gestation.

Akin to the situation with FVIIIc, both elevated FIXc and elevated fibrinogen levels are also associated with VTE. In the case of fibrinogen there is also a link with the development of arterial thrombosis.

Elevated FVIIIc, FIXc and fibrinogen levels and pregnancy outcome

As noted in Chapter 1, FVIIIc rises progressively with increasing gestation in normal pregnancies. Given this change, locally derived gestation-specific reference ranges are required before the impact of FVIIIc on pregnancy outcome can be assessed. Limited information suggests that FVIIIc levels (perhaps through the acquired aPCR phenotype) can have an influence on the development of PET. Further work is, however, required to determine if elevated early pregnancy FVIIIc, FIXc or fibrinogen levels carry any independent role in predicting pregnancy outcome.

Antiphospholipid syndrome (APS)

APS is defined as a combination of thrombosis and/or vascular complications of pregnancy that have occurred in the presence of persisting antibodies to negatively charged membrane phospholipids. It may occur as a primary syndrome or be a manifestation of systemic lupus erythematosus (SLE). However, it is becoming increasingly apparent that APS is a misnomer, as, in the majority of cases, it is not the binding of these antibodies to phospholipid but rather their binding to phospholipid-binding proteins (such as β2-glycoprotein-1, prothrombin, FV or protein C) that is important in their link with thrombosis.

Although individual assays, such as anti-β_2-glycoprotein-1 or anti-prothrombin antibody tests are available, most centers currently test for two forms of antiphospholipid activity: anticardiolipin antibodies (which can be detected by enzyme-linked immunosorbent assay (ELISA) and are of IgG, IgM or IgA class) and the presence of a lupus inhibitor (widely known as a lupus anticoagulant). It should be noted that the ELISA tests for anticardiolipin antibodies require β_2-glycoprotein-1 to be present in the test kit for the great majority of antiphospholipid antibodies to be detected.

Although it appears increasingly likely that the actions of the lupus inhibitor are related to activity against a combination of phospholipid with either β_2-glycoprotein-1 or prothrombin, the lupus inhibitor is currently detected by the effect it has on clotting tests. To diagnose a lupus inhibitor the patient plasma (which has been spun to reduce the number of platelets present) should prolong a phospholipid-dependent clotting time. This is usually demonstrated on an APTT (see Chapter 1), with confirmation on another clotting test called the dilute Russell viper venom test (dRVVT). An inhibitor will increase both the APTT and the dRVVT. The diagnosis requires there to be a failure to correct this prolongation when the test is repeated, using a mixture of patient plasma and normal plasma. Finally, the assessment is complete if the test is corrected by the addition of frozen, thawed platelets (the freeze–thaw process exposes phospholipid which is normally expressed on the inner aspect of the platelet membrane) or the addition of another source of excess phospholipid. In all cases, the antibody activity should be shown to be persistent, with a positive repeat assessment seen 6–8 weeks after the initial evaluation.

The prevalence of antiphospholipid antibodies (either a lupus inhibitor or elevated levels of anticardiolipin antibodies) can be detected in 2–12% of women of childbearing age, but may be of higher prevalence in those with a history of arterial thrombosis, venous thrombosis or fetal loss. The exact relationship of anticardiolipin antibodies to vascular disease is clouded by a number of issues: the large number of assays available; the ongoing debate regarding the relevance of antibodies of IgM or IgA class; the variations in the cut-off used for reporting abnormal results and; the difference in the quantity of β_2-glycoprotein-1 in each ELISA assay.

The physiological function of β_2-glycoprotein-1 is not clear, although β_2-glyco-protein-1 antibodies appear capable of counteracting the effects of TF pathway inhibitor and can also affect the effect of aPC on FVa. Thus, by a variety of actions, the mixture of detectable antiphospholipid antibodies can act to cause either direct endothelial activation and oxidative injury, or to activate coagulation through proteins such as prothrombin, FV and protein C or β_2-glycoprotein-1. In addition, binding of these antibodies to placental trophoblast may contribute to alteration in implantation and pregnancy failure.

APS and pregnancy outcome

The presence of persisting antiphospholipid antibodies is associated with placental infarction, and such antibodies are more often found in those with fetal loss occurring after 10 weeks gestation (i.e. fetal rather than embryonic or pre-embryonic loss), PET, IUGR, VTE and arterial thrombosis. Indeed, it has been estimated that up to 20% of women with antiphospholipid antibodies will have

Table 7.5 – Management options for antiphospholipid syndrome (APS) in pregnancy

Consider past pregnancy outcome
Confirm ACA/ lupus inhibitor status
Manage systemic lupus erythematosis (SLE), (If present)
Use low dose aspirin, when pregnancy confirmed (benefits may be limited to those with multiple fetal losses)
If previous venous thromboembolism (VTE), consider thromboprophylaxis (see Chapter 6)
Uterine artery Doppler 20–24 weeks may have value in risk of PET IUGR
If high PET risk, monitor urine and blood pressure
Corticosteroids, no evidence of benefit
Intravenous immunoglobulin, no evidence for overall benefit
Vitamin C/E supplementation, consider only if high risk PET
Low-molecular-weight heparin (LMWH) + aspirin, antenatal: consider risk:benefit ratio if ≥3 losses,
Puerperium: only LMWH if required for thromboprophylaxis

ACA, Anticardiolipin antibody; IUGR, Intrauterine growth restriction; PET, Pre-eclampsia.

obstetrics complications. Of these, the most precise information comes from those with a lupus inhibitor, which carries between a 3.0- and 4.8-fold risk of obstetric complications, although it is more likely to be associated with fetal loss in subjects who have SLE.

There is, however, a great variation in risk, which seems more dependent on the maternal obstetric history rather than on the presence, or absence, of detectable antiphospholipid activity. Given this variation in risk, the ability to use these tests to usefully predict pregnancy-associated disorders, especially in primigravid subjects, or in those in whom the antibody is an incidental finding, is far from certain. The management of APS in pregnancy requires an individual assessment, but the potential options are considered (Table 7.5).

References

Poort SR, Rosendaal FR, Reitsma PH, Bertina RM. A common genetic variation in the 3′–untranslated region of the prothrombin gene is associated with elevated plasma prothrombin levels and an increase in venous thrombosis. Blood 1996; 88(10): 3698–703.

CHAPTER 8
Thrombocytopenia in pregnancy

Maternal thrombocytopenia is commonly found in pregnancy. This is usually due to physiological changes with increasing gestation (termed gestational thrombocytopenia), or is caused by idiopathic thrombocytopenic purpura (ITP). Thrombocytopenia also occurs in association with a wide variety of both pregnancy-associated and non-pregnancy-associated conditions (Table 8.1).

Gestational thrombocytopenia

Towards the end of pregnancy at least 5% of women have a platelet count below the usual non-pregnant reference range $(150-400 \times 10^9/1)$. Although this gestational thrombocytopenia can be difficult to distinguish from ITP, the platelet count is seldom $<80 \times 10^9/1$ (although counts as low as $50 \times 10^9/1$ without significant disease have occasionally been reported). Thus, the diagnosis of gestational thrombocytopenia is most often made in the third trimester. It is con-

Table 8.1 – Thrombocytopenia in pregnancy

Spurious (i.e. clumping or poor sampling)
Gestational
Immune thrombocytopenic purpura (ITP)
Heparin-induced thrombocytopenia (HIT)
Post-transfusion purpura (PTP)
Acute Fatty Liver of Pregnancy
Pre-eclampsia (PET)/ hemolysis, elevated liver enzymes, and low platelets (HELLP) syndrome
Thrombotic thrombocytopenic purpura (TTP)/ Hemolytic uremic syndrome (HUS)
Disseminated intravascular coagulation (DIC)
Drug-induced thrombocytopenia
Systemic lupus erythematosis (SLE)/antiphospholipid syndrome (APAS)
Viral (HIV, Epstein-Barr virus (EBV), cytomegalovirus (CMV))
Congenital thrombocythemias/thrombocytopenia
Hypersplenism
Type IIb von Willebrand's disease (vWD)
Marrow dysfunction/hematinic deficiency

sidered that gestational thrombocytopenia is not the result of an immune disorder, but is due to a combination of hemodilution and a physiological increase in platelet clearance, with gestational thrombocytopenia representing the extreme end of the physiological reduction in platelet count which occurs in most normal pregnancies. Gestational thrombocytopenia does not cause maternal or fetal problems. In particular, fetal thrombocytopenia is no more common in such pregnancies than it is in women with normal platelet counts (in whom around 4% will have a baby with mild thrombocytopenia). If the platelet count is $>80 \times 10^9/l$, there are no implications for pregnancy management and it will resolve after delivery.

Diagnosis of gestational thrombocytopenia

A diagnosis of gestational thrombocytopenia requires exclusion of the other causes of thrombocytopenia (see Table 8.1), but this condition accounts for almost 75% of cases of thrombocytopenia diagnosed in pregnancy.

All patients presenting with significant thrombocytopenia ($<100 \times 10^9/l$) should have a blood film examined for evidence of platelet clumping, which indicates a factitious thrombocytopenia. In particular, in around 0.1% of adults, EDTA (which is used as a sample anticoagulant) can lead to an EDTA-dependent platelet agglutination causing a spuriously low platelet count. The blood film should also be examined for red cell fragmentation (indicating microangiopathic hemolytic anemia – MAHA), leukemia, myelodysplasia and megaloblastic anemia.

The platelet count in early pregnancy should be reviewed, as this will be normal in gestational thrombocytopenia. Such individuals also require investigation of folic acid status, renal and liver function, a coagulation screen and exclusion of autoimmune disorders such as antiphospholipid antibody syndrome (APAS), systemic lupus erythematosis (SLE) and HIV infection (Table 8.2).

In addition, pregnancy complications, particularly pre-eclampsia (including hemolysis, elevated liver enzymes, and low platelets (HELLP) syndrome), should be considered and, rarely, a coincidental diagnosis of thrombotic thrombocytopenic purpura (TTP) and hemolytic uremic syndrome (HUS) may be made

Table 8.2 – Investigation of thrombocytopenia in pregnancy

Blood film to exclude platelet clumps, microangiopathic hemolytic anemia (MAHA) or other hematological disorders
Coagulation screen (to include fibrinogen and D-dimer levels)
Renal and liver function tests
Antiphospholipid antibodies
Anti-DNA antibodies to exclude systemic lupus erythematosis (SLE) (ANA is sufficient as a screening test)

ANA, Ante-nuclear antigen

(Table 8.3). However, the main differential diagnosis is usually ITP or pre-eclampsia, which account for around 4 and 21%, respectively, of cases of pregnancy thrombocytopenia. Clearly, it may be impossible to be certain that the diagnosis is gestational thrombocytopenia rather than ITP, and in this situation it is best to err on the side of caution and use the same precautions as in ITP to minimize the risk of hemorrhagic complications in the baby (see Table 8.4).

Table 8.3 – Differential diagnosis of thrombocytopenia in pregnancy

	Incidence	Typical gestation at diagnosis	Associated features	Worst platelet count ($\times 10^9$/l)
Gestational	5–7 in 100	Second to third trimester	Blood pressure (BP) √ Blood film √	<100
Pre-eclampsia (PET) hemolysis, elevated liver enzymes, and low platelets (HELLP)	2 in 100	Late second to third trimester	BP ↑ Proteinuria MAHA Uric acid ↑ LFT ↑ ±Antithrombin ↓	Variable (with disease severity)
Idiopathic thrombocytopenic purpura (ITP)	<5 in 10 000	First trimester	BP √ Blood film √ ±Known ITP/AI history	<50
Acute fatty liver	1 in 10 000– 15 000	Third trimester	Cholestatic LFT ↑ Glucose ↓ Fibrinogen ↓ Antithrombin ↓	Variable (with disease severity)
Thrombotic thrombocytopenic purpura (TTP)/hemolytic uremic syndrome (HUS)	1 in 25 000	Second to third trimester/ postpartum	MAHA Renal ↓ or Neurological ↓ Coagulation ↑/√ antithrombin √	<20
Disseminated intravascular coagulation (DIC)	–	Second to third trimester/ postpartum	Coagulation √ Fibrinogen ↓ + underlying disorder (PET/abruption or major obstetric hemorrhage/ amniotic fluid embolus/ uterine rupture/sepsis/ retained fetus)	Variable (with disease severity)

AI, Auto immune; LFT, Liver function test

Table 8.4 – Gestational thrombocytopenia

Mild and asymptomatic occurs in 7% of pregnancies
Normal platelet count at booking
Occurs in third trimester
No fetal problem
Resolves after delivery
If platelets >80×10^9/l: no implications for pregnancy management
If unable to distinguish from idiopathic thrombocytopenic purpura (ITP), avoid fetal scalp electrode, fetal blood sampling, ventouse delivery and rotational forceps

Immune thrombocytopenic purpura (ITP)

ITP results in a platelet count of <150×10^9/l and is due to auto-antibody-mediated binding and destruction of platelets by the reticuloendothelial system. The autoantibodies in ITP are generally directed against the platelet surface glycoprotein complexes IIb/IIIa or Ib/IX. Immune-mediated thrombocytopenia can also be caused by allogenic antiplatelet antibodies which lead to post-transfusion purpura (PTP), neonatal alloimmune thrombocytopenia (NAIT) and heparin-induced thrombocytopenia (HIT) (Table 8.5).

Autoantiplatelet antibodies can occur in association with drugs, SLE, rheumatoid arthritis, HIV and lymphoma. Recently, eradication of *Helicobacter pylori* has been shown to be of benefit in some subjects with ITP, although the causal mechanism, or the role of such therapy in pregnancy, is not known (Table 8.6). Nonetheless, a breath test or serological assessment to detect *H pylori* may be worthwhile, especially in refractory cases.

As the antiplatelet antibodies cross the placenta the baby may become thrombocytopenic, with around 9–15% having thrombocyopenia and up to 1.5% developing an intracranial hemorrhage.

Table 8.5 – Disorders associated with immune-mediated thrombocytopenia

Helicobacter pylori
Systemic lupus erythematosis (SLE)
Lymphoma chronic lymphatic leukemia (CLL)
Heparin-induced thrombocytopenia (HIT)
HIV
Post-transfusion purpura (PTP)
Drugs

Table 8.6 – Experimental therapies in idiopathic thrombocytopenic purpura (ITP)

Intravenous Anti-RhD treatment

- Anti-RhD is usually used to prevent RhD alloimmunization
- In RhD-positive subjects, 50–70mg/kg anti-RhD increases platelets in <70%
- Side effects include headache, fever and a risk of hemolysis
- Anti-RhD results in less donor exposure than IVIgG
- Repeat dosing may be required
- The effect on the fetus requires more study
- Anti-RhD may have a role as a secondline therapy

Helicobacter eradication

- Gastric Helicobacter may be more common in ITP
- In refractory ITP consider screening for Helicobacter
- The benefits of eradication of Helicobacter in pregnancy is unknown

Diagnosis of ITP in pregnancy

Adult chronic ITP often affects women of childbearing age and is found in 1–5 in 10 000 pregnancies. In fact, it is not infrequently diagnosed for the first time during pregnancy. This is particularly so since the inclusion of routine platelet counting in the mechanical assessment of the blood count. The most likely presentation is as asymptomatic thrombocytopenia on routine blood count testing (Table 8.7). In addition, women known to have ITP may suffer an exacerbation during pregnancy, and occasionally a new diagnosis is heralded by severe symptomatic thrombocytopenia in pregnancy.

As in non-pregnant subjects, the diagnosis of ITP in pregnancy is one of exclusion of other disorders (see Tables 8.1 and 8.2). In general, if there are no additional clinical features, and the blood count and film are otherwise normal, bone

Table 8.7 – Features of thrombocytopenic purpura (ITP) in pregnancy

A low platelet count out-with pregnancy is invaluable in the diagnosis of ITP
ITP may be impossible to distinguish from gestational thrombocytopenia
Platelets $<100 \times 10^9$/l: screen for pre-eclampsia (PET), coagulopathy, autoimmune disease, HIV
No bone marrow examination unless a lymphoma is suspected, or a splenectomy is required
The bleeding time does not predict hemorrhage
Corticosteroids, intravenous human normal immunoglobulin (IVIgG) or splenectomy do not effect the fetal platelet count
The mode of delivery should be determined by obstetric indications
Neonatal alloimmune thrombocytopenia (NAIT) should be excluded in all neonates with thrombocytopenia and hemorrhage

marrow examination is not required to make the diagnosis of ITP in pregnancy. In addition, the measurement of maternal antiplatelet immunoglobulin or blood thrombopoietin levels are not valuable in the routine diagnosis of ITP in pregnancy.

Treatment of ITP

There have been few randomized clinical trials on the management of ITP in pregnancy. As it is very likely that the platelet count will continue to fall as pregnancy progresses (reaching a nadir in the third trimester), and as spontaneous bleeding problems are unlikely if the platelet count is $>20 \times 10^9/l$, the management of ITP in pregnancy is usually focused on achieving an adequate platelet count for delivery, in particular to allow neuraxial anesthesia, and to minimize the risk of fetal bleeding during labor and delivery.

The treatment options during pregnancy are similar to those used out-with pregnancy, with due regard to the presence of the fetus. In general, if the platelet count is $>20 \times 10^9/l$ and the patient is asymptomatic, then monitoring of the platelet count and of the patient for bleeding is all that is required. If, at delivery, the patient is asymptomatic then a spontaneous vaginal delivery or Cesarean section could take place if the platelet count is $>50 \times 10^9/l$ (uncomplicated vaginal delivery is probably safe at levels $>30-40 \times 10^9/l$, but as the risk of Cesarean section is present in every labor it is best to aim for at least a level of $50 \times 10^9/l$). If the patient requires epidural anesthesia then a platelet count of $>80 \times 10^9/l$ is recommended (Table 8.8). Following delivery, non-steroidal anti-inflammatory drugs (NSAID) should be avoided for postoperative analgesia unless the platelet count is $>100 \times 10^9/l$. It is also important to consider the woman's risk of venous thromboembolism (VTE), and for those considered at increased risk, graduated elastic compression stockings and/or low-molecular-weight heparin (LMWH) can be used. The latter is considered satisfactory if the platelet count is $>50 \times 10^9/l$, the patient has no hemorrhagic problems and has a significant risk of VTE.

Firstline therapies

There are two firstline options currently used. These are oral corticosteroids and intravenous human normal immunoglobulin (IVIgG). Both appear to have

Table 8.8 –Treatment of idiopathic thrombocytopenic purpura (ITP)

Platelet count $>20 \times 10^9/l$ and asymptomatic	Monitor until delivery
Platelet count $>40-50 \times 10^9/l$ and asymptomatic	Safe for normal vaginal delivery
Platelet count $>50 \times 10^9/l$ and asymptomatic	Safe for Cesarean section
Platelet count $>80 \times 10^9/l$ and asymptomatic	Safe for epidural anesthesia

similar response rates – around 70% of patients will respond to IVIgG, with a variable response rate for steroids, which is, at best, between 50 and 66%. Clinicians vary in their choice, with some preferring IVIgG. This is most often due to the perceived side effects of oral corticosteroids, although such side effects are not usually critical with a short duration of high-dose steroids used in anticipation of delivery. The cost of IVIgG and, more importantly, the fact that it is a human blood product must also be considered. (Table 8.9). In general, if treatment is to be required for a short time, then corticosteroids are a useful option at a dose of prednisolone of 1mg/kg/day in the first instance, continued for 2–4 weeks then tailing off the dose. If the duration of therapy is likely to be longer (treatment starting in the first or second trimester), then IVIgG, at a dose of 0.4g/kg/day for 5 days or 1g/kg/day for 2 days, has been used with an equivalent response rate evident in at least one randomized trial. However, depending on the product (see Chapter 2), there may be a higher risk of renal impairment with the more intense schedule, and the first schedule is to be preferred if there are pre-existing fluid balance problems or renal impairment. IVIgG most often results in a response of 2–3 weeks duration and repeat dosing may be required if a continuing hemostatic challenge is anticipated.

The mechanism of action of IVIg in ITP is largely unknown, but it may involve the blockade of Fc receptors on macrophages and other effectors of antibody-dependent cytotoxicity, or be due to the presence of anti-idiotype antibodies in IVIgG which block autoantibody binding to circulating platelets. IVIgG may also block Fc receptors on the placenta and so may prevent transfer of maternal antiplatelet antibody but this is unproven in practice and remains a theoretical benefit of IVIgG.

Secondline therapies

This includes high-dose methylprednisolone (1000mg) or azathioprine, which is satisfactory for use in pregnancy, or a combination of these therapies with IVIgG. Obviously, danazol, vinca alkaloids and cyclophosphamide are not suitable for the pregnant patient. For patients who do not respond to conventional second-line therapies, anti-RhD immunoglobulin (see Table 8.6), and even interferon and mycophenolate mofetil or retuximab could be considered, but experience, even in the non-pregnant, is very limited.

Splenectomy is best avoided in pregnancy, but, if considered essential, is best carried out between 13 and 20 weeks gestation. At present, the role of laproscopic splenectomy in pregnancy is not known. In 66% of non-pregnant subjects, splenectomy will result in a normal platelet count. A number of studies have suggested that the patient's response to IVIgG may predict the response to splenectomy. However, it is not known if this has any predictive value in pregnancy. The use of indium-labeled autologous platelet scanning to identify whether the platelet destruction is splenic, hepatic or diffuse would not be a favored option in pregnant subjects. This test is, however, the most sensitive pre-

Table 8.9 – Treatment and outcome of thrombocytopenia in pregnancy

	Mechanism	Treatment	Treatment complications	Maternal outcome	Fetal testing	Fetal outcomes	Recur
Gestational	Hemodilution Clearance ↑	Not required	–	√	None	Platelet (Plat) <150, 4%	Yes
Idiopathic thrombocytopenic purpura (ITP)	Autoantibodies	Corticosteroids Immunoglobulin Azothioprine Splenectomy	Weight ↑, blood pressure (BP) ↑, glucose ↑ Allergy. fluid ↑, urea ↑, Infection transmission ? Miscarriage/thrombosis/ infection	√ or Hemorrhage	Full blood count (FBC) Day 1–5	Well 90% Plat<50, <20% Intra cerebral hemorrhage (ICH) <1.5% Mortality 0.6%	Yes
Pre-eclampsia (PET) hemolysis, elevated liver enzymes, and low platelets (HELLP)	Platelet/endothelial activation	Supportive (±platelets/fresh frozen plasma (FFP)) Deliver	Allergy, fever, transmissible agents		FBC Day 1–5	None Platelets ↓ Intrauterine growth restriction (IUGR) Abortion	Yes
Thrombotic thrombo-cytopenic purpura (TTP)/hemolytic uremic syndrome (HUS)	↓ ADAMTS–13	Plasma exchange ±FFP	Fluid imbalance, BP ↓ Allergy, fever, transmissible agents	Mortality 10–30%	–		Yes
Acute fatty liver	? Long chain fatty acid deficiency (LCHAD) ↓	Glucose Fluid balance General support Liver transplant ±platelets/FFP/ Cryoprecipitate (cryo)	Allergy, fever, transmissible agents	Mortality 5–20%		Mortality <15%	?Yes
Disseminated intravascular coagulation (DIC)	Consumption	Treat cause ±platelets/FFP/cryo	Allergy, fever, transmissible agents	Depends on etiology	–	Variable	No

Table 8.10 – Preventing post-splenectomy infection

At least 2 weeks prior to splenectomy

- Polyvalent Pneumococcal vaccine (Pneumovax II)
- Hemophilus influenza B vaccine (Hib)
- Meningococcal C vaccine (Men C)

Following splenectomy

- Phenoxymethylpenicillin (250–500mg bd) or erythromycin (500mg od)*
- Annual influenza vaccine
- Antimalarial prophylaxis when appropriate
- Anticoagulant prophylaxis when appropriate

*The required duration is not yet known but may be lifelong.

dictor of response to splenectomy, by identifying those patients where splenic destruction is present.

As with non-pregnant subjects, the removal of the spleen leads to a lifelong increased risk of infection, predominantly with capsulated organisms (Table 8.10). Splenectomy also results in a lifelong thrombotic tendency. Although the mechanism of this is not understood, it may relate to circulating nucleated red cells (which are seen in the blood after splenectomy), or be due to the loss of splenic regulation of white cell and platelet counts. In any event, this must be considered when assessing the patient risk factors for thrombosis and thrombo-prophylaxis.

Management of delivery in ITP

The baby's platelet count cannot be reliably predicted from either the mother's platelet count, maternal antiplatelet immunoglobulin levels, or by the presence (or absence) of the spleen. Fetal blood sampling by cordocentesis carries a mortality similar to that of the risk of intracerebral hemorrhage (see Table 8.9), and scalp blood sampling is prone to spurious low results (due to clotting of the blood sample) and may itself cause significant hemorrhage. Thus, as the status of the baby cannot be determined antenatally, procedures at delivery that would pose an additional bleeding risk (particularly of intracranial hemorrhage) should be avoided. There is no evidence that Cesarean section is safer for the thrombocytopenic fetus than an uncomplicated vaginal delivery and, in any case, the maximum fall in the platelet count in the newborn is likely to occur some 24–48 hours after delivery. Fetal scalp electrodes and fetal blood samples are best avoided, and if an assisted vaginal delivery is required, ventouse should be avoided as this can cause severe scalp hematoma. Rotational forceps are also best avoided due to risk of intracranial bleeding if the baby is affected, but a straight-forward mid- or low-cavity forceps delivery would be considered appropriate, if required. At delivery, a cord platelet count should be determined in all babies whose mother has been diagnosed with ITP. Close monitoring is required over the next 2–5 days. In children with evidence of bleeding, or a platelet count $<20 \times 10^9/l$, IVIgG (at 1g/kg) produces a rapid response. Neonatal life-threatening hemorrhage may also require platelet transfusion.

Autoimmune neutropenia (AIN)

In parallel with ITP, AIN also occurs, and a number of cases of AIN in pregnancy have also been reported. There is, however, very little information on pregnancy-specific management. However, the genetically engineered granulocyte colony-stimulating factor (G-CSF) has been used, with some success, to increase the production and release of neutrophils in subjects who have an autoantibody to their own neutrophils. In subjects on G-CSF who become pregnant, the G-CSF is often witheld antepartum, as the effects on the fetus are not known. The passive placental transfer of antibodies can result in neutropenia in the neonate, and very limited evidence suggests that G-CSF, given in the final trimester, may have a beneficial effect on the neonatal neutrophil count (either by increasing maternal neutrophils and reducing free maternal antibody, or by stimulation of neutrophil release in the fetus). However, whether this is a safe approach, and whether maternal autoantibody titers, or the specificity of the antibody in the mother will assist in the prediction of the neonatal blood count, requires further invesigation. G-CSF is, however, probably safe in nursing mothers. Although it does cross the breast, limted evidence suggests that it causes a local, but not systemic effect, in the neonate.

Thrombotic thrombocytopenic purpura (TTP)/hemolytic uremic syndrome (HUS)

TTP and HUS are characterized by a low platelet count, red cell fragmentation (resulting in MAHA: see above) and multi-organ failure. It is usually considered that TTP is more often associated with neurological abnormalities and non-renal organ ischemia, whilst patients with HUS have predominantly renal manifestations. However, as there is a significant cross-over in symptomatology, it is often difficult to distinguish between these two conditions clinically.

TTP occurs most often as an idopathic syndrome and, interestingly, the incidence of TTP is increasing in the Western world; this may be due to cases precipitated by drug exposure. Although it can occur as a congenital form, which may recur, around 66% of adult cases are non-recurrent. TTP also occurs secondary to pregnancy, drugs such as clopidogrel, ticlopidine, tacrolimus, the combined contraceptive pill, bone marrow transplant, SLE, malignancy and infection with HIV or Escherichia coli-0157. As with TTP, HUS may be precipitated by pregnancy, follow infection with cytotoxin-producing serotypes of organisms such as *E Coli* or Shigella, or follow administration of drugs such as cyclosporine, quinine and chemotherapeutic agents.

The endothelium releases ultralarge multimers of von Willebrand Factor (vWF), which are subsequently cleaved by the metalloprotease ADAMTS-13 (A disintegrin and metalloproteinase with thrombospondin domains, number 13) in the plasma. This results in the circulation of the correct balance of vWF multimers and TTP/HUS is characterized by a failure of cleavage of these multimers. As noted above, in TTP, this can be due to a congenital deficiency of the cleavage enzyme, but is more commonly due to acquired autoantibody formation. However, in HUS, and in many cases of TTP, the vWF cleaving activity is normal. In the rare patients with recurrent or familial HUS, there is an abnormally low level of the complement control protein Factor H, with overactivity of complement component 3 whenever the alternative complement pathway is activated.

Just as insufficient vWF multimers lead to bleeding through a reduction in platelet aggregation (see Chapter 4), an excess of circulating ultralarge multimers results in an increase in platelet aggregation and platelet consumption, which leads to microvascular platelet thrombi (with little fibrin, but an abundance of vWF in the platelet thrombi formed) as well as endothelial apoptosis and MAHA. This results in downstream ischemia and infarction in organ systems.

There are many reasons why pregnancy may pre-dispose to TTP/HUS. As detailed in Chapter 1, normal pregnancy is associated with an increase in Factor (F) VIIc, FVIIIc, FIXc, vWF and thrombin generation, as well as a reduction in protein S. These physiological changes may result in hypercoagulability and exacerbate any predisposition to TTP or HUS. Indeed, thrombophilic risk factors such as FV Leiden and obesity have also been linked with the occurrence of TTP. More particularly, pregnancy is often the precipitant for recurrent episodes of TTP that occur in subjects with the rare congenital deficiency of ADAMTS-13. There is also evidence that there is a 30% reduction in ADAMTS-13 in normal pregnancy and that the pregnancy level of ADAMTS-13 is inversely related to vWF levels. If there is a congenital deficiency, a further reduction may be seen in normal pregnancy. As noted above, TTP can, however, occur with no evident in reduction in ADAMTS-13 activity, and reduction in ADAMTS-13 itself is not specific to TTP/HUS.

Diagnosis of TTP/HUS in pregnancy

With regard to HUS in pregnancy, the presentation is typically a single episode (almost always postpartum) with the classic triad of thrombocytopenia, hemolysis, and renal failure. It can accompany HELLP syndrome, where the liver dysfunction is more marked (see Table 8.3). While TTP should present with the classic pentad of fever, hemolysis, thrombocytopenia, central nervous system (CNS) signs and renal dysfunction (proteinuria/hematuria), all five are only

Table 8.11 – Investigation of suspected TTP/HUS during pregnancy.

FBC/Film
Reticulocyte count
Coagulation screen
Urea and electrolytes
LFT
LDH
Coomb's test
Urinalysis

FBC, Full blood count; LDH, Lactate dehydrogenase; LFT, Liver function tests

present in around 50% of cases. The CNS signs, thrombocytopenia and hemolysis are, however, more marked than with PET or HUS, but the hypertension may not be severe (Table 8.12). TTP, particularly recurrent TTP, usually presents before 24 weeks of pregnancy and intrauterine growth restriction (IUGR) and fetal death is usual. As noted above, isolated episodes of TTP can occur and relapse is common in pregnancy.

Although routine clotting tests are often normal in the early stages of TTP/HUS, as the disease progresses there may be activation of coagulation and disseminated intravascular coagulation (DIC). However, the accompanying elevation of D-dimer levels may often be difficult to distinguish from the elevated D-dimer levels of normal pregnancy (see Chapter 1).

A comparison of the symptoms and investigations in thrombocytopenic disorders is shown (Table 8.3). It has been reported that plasma antithrombin levels may be of assistance in the distinction of PET/HELLP (reduced levels) from TTP/HUS (normal levels) (Table 8.3). However, reduced and normal levels may be seen in either condition, and establishing a reduced level requires a local pregnancy-related reference range.

Table 8.12 – TTP/HUS or PET/HELLP.

Significant anemia and microangiopathic hemolytic anemia (MAHA) points to TTP/HUS
Severe hypertension points more to PET/HELLP than TTP/HUS
Severe renal or central nervous system (CNS) disease points more to TTP/HUS than PET/HELLP
Fever is unusual in HELLP
Often delivery leads to resolution of PET/HELLP, but a transient deterioration may occur
TTP is not improved by delivery and often PET/HELLP and TTP/HUS are only distinguished after delivery

Treatment of TTP/HUS

With perhaps the exception of bacterial endotoxin-related HUS (where supportive care is the main aspect of therapy) and recurrent or congenital TTP (see below), it is unlikely that a clear distinction between the two syndromes of TTP and HUS will be possible in the majority of pregnancy-related cases. As a consequence, both will be considered predominantly as a single syndrome when considering therapy, particularly as there may be benefit in plasma exchange in non-toxin-related HUS (Table 8.13).

Firstline therapies

The mainstay of treatment of TTP/HUS is plasma exchange, which removes the large vWF multimers and autoantibodies, and supplements the vWF cleaving enzymes. This has produced a remarkable reduction in the mortality of this condition. The treatment schedules used in pregnancy are derived from those used in non-pregnant subjects. Plasma exchange should be instituted within 24 hours of presentation, as this has a bearing on prognosis, and subjects should be managed in a facility that can provide an uninterrupted service. The optimal number of plasma exchange procedures required is not known, but most authorities recommend that there should be a further two procedures after complete clinical remission. Indeed, many facilities would taper off the exchanges rather than stopping them abruptly, even after these two further procedures. Similarly, the optimal exchange regime has not been determined, and either daily exchanges of 1 or 1.5 plasma volumes for the first 3 days followed by 1 plasma volume thereafter have both been used to good effect.

In addition, the optimum fluid replacement has not yet been ascertained. Fresh frozen plasma (FFP) is the standard therapy in most countries. However, cryosupernatant may offer some advantages over FFP. Cryosupernatant is derived from the manufacture of cryoprecipitate and contains lesser amounts of the larger vWF multimers, but may not be widely available. In view of the potential risk of viral contamination of FFP, solvent detergent-treated FFP (SD-FFP) can

Table 8.13 – Thrombotic thrombocytopenic purpura (TTP)/hemolytic uremic syndrome (HUS)

Daily plasma exchange as soon as possible
Fresh frozen plasma infusion if delay in plasma exchange
Consider corticosteroids and aspirin
Consider refractory if deterioration or no response in 7 days
If refractory, change replacement fluid or increase exchange frequency
Anaphylaxis to plasma exchange may occur in <1 in 400
If febrile, check for underlying infection

also be used as the fluid replacement in plasma exchange. SD-FFP contains lesser amounts of the larger vWF multimers, and may also carry a lesser risk of adverse reactions, than standard FFP.

When plasma exchange is not immediately available, FFP infusion (at 30ml/kg), with due attention to the risks of fluid overload, may be beneficial whilst exchange is being organized. In the rare congenital TTP with deficiency of the cleaving metalloproteinases, exchange may not be required and FFP infusion alone may be sufficient to induce remission.

Additional therapies

Any agent that could have precipitated TTP, such as clopidogrel, should be stopped. As an immunoglobulin-mediated reduction in ADAMTS-13 activity occurs in association with TTP, intravenous methylprednisolone has been used as an adjunct to plasma exchange, although the benefit:risk ratio of this approach in pregnancy has not been formally assessed. However, there is no specific contraindication to corticosteroid use in this situation.

Similarly, as many of the effects of TTP may be mediated through platelet activation, the use of antiplatelet agents is an attractive option. In this regard, there may be some benefit in the empirical addition of aspirin to the plasma exchange regime when the platelet count is restored to $>50 \times 10^9/l$. Use of aspirin when the patient is severely thrombocytopenic can, however, precipitate hemorrhagic complications.

All patients should receive folic acid and be vaccinated (when the platelet count allows) against hepatitis B. Red cell transfusion should be given according to clinical need, but platelet transfusions should be avoided in TTP. As with other conditions associated with thrombosis, there may be a role for thromboprophylaxis with LMWH, although the use of this requires an individual assessment of the relative bleeding/thrombosis risk.

Secondline therapies

The patient is regarded as being in remission if there is a resolution of neurological symptoms, the platelet count has normalized, the lactate dehydrogenase (LDH) has reduced to within reference limits and the hemoglobin is rising. Refractory disease would be defined as a failure of this after seven exchanges. If the patient deteriorates, or does not respond to the initial plasma exchange regime, a change to a higher plasma volume exchange (1.5 plasma volumes), a higher frequency (12 hourly) or a different replacement fluid (cryosupernatant or SD-FFP rather than standard FFP) has been recommended. The use of other immunosupressive therapies such as vincristine, cyclophosphamide and cyclosporine would be problematic whilst there is still a viable fetus and their use in pregnancy would be on a case-by-case basis. Generally, if the patient has reached this stage, she will usually have been delivered in either the maternal or fetal interest, or have suffered an intrauterine death.

Pre-eclampsia (PET)/hemolysis, elevated liver enzymes, and low platelets (HELLP) syndrome

PET is a hypertensive disorder that occurs in 3–6% of pregnancies and is most commonly seen in primigravid women, or more particularly in 'first-partner' pregnancies (see Chapter 7). The disease has varying severity from mild hypertension to severe hypertension with seizures, and can occur in the context of HELLP syndrome (Table 8.14). As detailed in Chapter 7, the cause of this disorder remains enigmatic, although it is undoubtedly related to abnormal placental trophoblast development early in pregnancy. This may relate to immune maladaption, placental ischemia, lipid-related oxidative stress or excess thrombogenesis.

Thrombocytopenia occurs in around half of subjects with PET and is most likely due to a combination of excess thrombin generation and endothelial activation. These prothrombotic changes result in an increase in activation, binding and clearance of platelets. Certainly, in the majority of subjects, the degree of thrombocytopenia is linked to the clinical severity of the PET.

Diagnosis of PET and HELLP

See Chapter 7.

Table 8.14 – Hemolysis, elevated liver enzymes, and low platelets (HELLP) summary

Hemolysis: schistocytes and LDH >600U/l
Elevated liver enzymes (AST >70U/l)
Low platelets (<100 × 10^9/l) with subclassification based upon count
Coagulation tests (activated partial thromboplastin time (APTT) and prothrombin time (PT)) remain normal, but sensitive tests of coagulation consistent with low-grade disseminated intravascular coagulation (DIC))
Liver shows periportal hemorrhage, necrosis, fibrin deposition and steatosis (overlap with acute fatty liver of pregnancy (AFLP))
Thirty-three per cent occur postpartum
In severe pre-eclampsia (PET), 6% have one of the HELLP criteria, 12% have two, and 10% have all criteria
HELLP presentation is non-specific with malaise, but RUQ pain and edema are common clinical features: 50% are normotensive and >6% do not have proteinuria at diagnosis
Management: delivery and supportive therapy with steroids
HELLP outcome in next pregnancy:
HELLP in 3%
PET in 19%
Intrauterine growth restriction (IUGR) in 12%

IU/l, International units/liter; LDH, Lactate dehydrogenase; RUQ, right upper quadrant; U/l, Units/liter

Treatment of PET/HELLP syndrome

The treatment of PET/HELLP is geared towards stabilization of the mother. This requires the control of blood pressure, which allows the pregnancy to proceed and reduces the need for medical intervention, although this does not appear to alter the course of the disease. Indeed, delivery is the only cure for PET. To control hypertension, the drug of choice is methyldopa, as there is a considerable experience of the use of this drug in pregnancy. A suitable alternative is labetolol. More acute blood pressure reduction may require labetolol, nifedipine or hydralazine. Fluid balance should be stabilized, but diuretics should be avoided, unless required for cardiac failure. There is also the need to consider seizure prophylaxis in fulminant disease and to achieve sufficient fetal maturation for delivery. When blood pressure is uncontrolled, hematological and biochemical parameters are deteriorating, or the patient is becoming symptomatic, delivery is indicated. This is particularly so when the pregnancy is beyond 34 weeks, but when it is between 24 and 34 weeks, the risks to the fetus of early delivery and the risk to the mother of the continuing pregnancy have to be balanced in determining the appropriate action. Following delivery, the disease process will resolve, but the systemic manifestations may worsen in the immediate postpartum period.

Symptomatic thrombocytopenia and the preparation for delivery may require platelet transfusion. In such patients, platelets may fail to achieve the expected increment due to platelet consumption, and the platelet count should be checked after dosing to confirm an adequate response. The platelet count may continue to fall after delivery, although in the majority of subjects delivery brings about a resolution of the disorder. For those with persisting thrombocytopenia and/or MAHA (indicating progressive disease after delivery), both plasma exchange and corticosteroids have been used to assist recovery. Any associated coagulopathy will require FFP. Hypofibrinogenemia is not common and, indeed, may be difficult to define given the substantial rise in fibrinogen seen with increasing gestation. If present, however, it may require specific treatment with cryoprecipitate or fibrinogen concentrate.

Acute fatty liver of pregnancy (AFLP)

AFLP is an unusual condition (complicating 1 in 10 000–15 000 pregnancies) that results from fatty infiltration of the liver and other organs during pregnancy. It is more common in obese subjects, in those with a multiple pregnancy and in those carrying a male fetus. It often presents with jaundice, which can rapidly progress to coagulopathy, hepatic failure and both fetal and maternal death. In 50% of subjects there may be associated features suggestive of PET, and in 20% of subjects features suggestive of HELLP syndrome. The condition has been reported to carry a maternal mortality risk of 5–20% and a fetal mortality risk of up to 15%.

Diagnosis of AFLP

The diagnosis of AFLP is suspected by a combination of clinical features (see Table 8.3). In particular, the detection in the third trimester, of a cholestatic pattern of liver function tests (LFTs), hypoglycemia and features of failure of synthetic hepatic function (e.g. hypofibrinogenemia and a reduction in plasma antithrombin levels) are suggestive of the disorder. The disease may be difficult to distinguish from PET/HELLP and will require the exclusion of other causes of hepatitis and confirmation of fatty infiltration in the liver by ultrasonography or magnetic resonance imaging (MRI). In general, when compared to HELLP syndrome, AFLP is more likely to be associated with higher serum levels of aspartate transaminase (AST) and hypoglycemia, and is more often accompanied by marked hyperuricemia, DIC and leukocytosis. The combination of these features will lead to a diagnosis in the majority of cases without the need for liver biopsy.

A potential causative mechanism is suggested by the link between AFLP and the carriage of a fetus with an inborn error of metabolism (resulting in a failure to oxidize long-chain fatty acids). Oxidation of fatty acids requires adequate function of mictochondrial trifunctional protein (MTP). MTP is coded by chromosome 2 and consists of three enzymes that carry out consecutive oxidation of free fatty acids. Free fatty acid metabolism is used to generate glucose and eventually adenosine triphosphate (ATP). In the absence of free fatty acid metabolism and inadequate glucose, a hypoglycemic lactic acidosis occurs, which is accompanied by infiltration (by abnormal lipids) of the liver, skeletal muscle, myocardium, kidney, pancreas and lungs.

A number of cases of acute fatty liver of pregnancy have been associated with the presence of fetal homozygous deficiency of one, or all three, of the components of the MTP. However, how alterations in placental free fatty acid metabolites lead to maternal disease is unknown, and further work is required to determine the exact contribution of inborn errors of fatty acid oxidation to the development of AFLP as well as PET/HELLP syndrome.

Treatment of AFLP

Treatment is aimed towards biochemical correction of hypoglycemia and fluid balance, correction of any associated renal insufficiency, coagulopathy, hypertension, concomitant sepsis and preparation for delivery. Severe hepatic failure may require the use of liver transplantation. It is known for AFLP to recur in subsequent pregnancies, but the exact incidence is hard to estimate. This may be due to the substantial mortality associated with the condition and the natural reluctance of some survivors to undertake a further pregnancy.

Heparin-induced thrombocytopenia (HIT)

HIT arises from the development of specific heparin-dependent IgG antibodies and should be considered in the differential diagnosis of thrombocytopenia for those receiving heparin in pregnancy. As detailed in Chapter 5, HIT commonly occurs after 5 days of therapy and is associated with a high risk of severe thrombosis due to platelet activation.

Diagnosis of HIT

A variety of tests to determine the presence of antibodies against the combined heparin-platelet Factor 4 antigen are employed. These are often based on enzyme-linked iummunosorbent assay (ELISA) technology or platelet function testing. The principal difficulty with these assays is the lack of standardization, and often the lack of information about their sensitivity and specificity for HIT. Because of this the diagnosis of HIT should remain principally a clinical one.

Treatment of HIT in pregnancy

For treatment options see Chapter 5.

Post-transfusion purpura (PTP)

PTP is a rare disorder (<1 in 5 million of Caucasian populations/year), although around 2% of female Caucasians may be at risk. It is most often seen in multiparous females, and although acute PTP is most likely after transfusion for postpartum hemorrhage, it should be considered in the differential diagnosis of thrombocytopenia if there has been an antenatal transfusion (see Chapter 2).

PTP has similarities to NAIT, although there are no reports of maternal thrombocytopenia in NAIT. Furthermore, the fetal thrombocytopenia in NAIT occurs because the fetus is positive for the corresponding antigen target of the IgG antibody transferred from the mother, whereas in PTP the platelet destruction occurs despite the mother being negative for the target platelet antigen. The development of the antibody in PTP is not invariable and is more common in subjects carrying human leukocyte antigen (HLA) DR3 (specifically DRw52). Although after acute PTP recurrence is possible, this is difficult to predict as there may be a period when further exposure to the human platelet antigen (HPA) will not elicit an anamnestic response.

Prevention of PTP

Effective prevention in pregnancy would require universal screening to determine the HPA phenotype of pregnant women, as well as the presence of existing maternal anti-HPA antibodies. It would also be necessary to supply appropriate antigen-negative blood throughout pregnancy. At present, it would seem unlikely that universal screening would be either cost or clinically effective. However, as noted in Chapter 2, subjects already known to have such antibodies should be transfused with appropriate HPA antigen-negative blood.

Treatment of PTP

For treatment options see Chapter 2.

Disseminated intravascular coagulation (DIC)

DIC has been defined as an 'acquired' syndrome, characterized by intravascular activation of coagulation with loss of localization, arising from different causes. It can originate from and cause damage to the microvasculature, which, if sufficiently severe, can produce organ dysfunction. The activation of coagulation leads to thrombin generation, consumption of clotting factors and anticoagulants, and the development of MAHA. This can lead to widespread thrombosis, bleeding and multi-organ failure.

DIC occurs in response to a wide variety of disorders (Table 8.15). In sepsis, the trigger may be the activation of cytokines, which leads to coagulation activation. DIC may also occur in response to the release of pro-coagulant material, such as fat, phospholipids, tissue factor and amniotic fluid. Such release is found in association with mismatched blood transfusions, obstetric complications or malignancy. DIC should be distinguished from other causes of MAHA, such as HUS and TTP.

Diagnosis of DIC in pregnancy

DIC is diagnosed when there is consumption of coagulation factors, as seen by:

- A prolonged prothrombin time (PT);
- A prolonged activated partial thromboplastin time (APTT);
- A reduction in fibrinogen;
- Evidence of an increase in fibrinolysis as shown by an increase in measurable fibrin degradation products, i.e. FDP, or more specifically D-dimers (see Chapter 1).

Table 8.15 – Causes of disseminated intravascular coagulation (DIC)

Sepsis
Major trauma
Placental abruption
Amniotic fluid emboli
Mismatched transfusion
Hepatic failure
Malignancy
Pancreatitis

In addition, there may also be a reduction in plasma antithrombin (due to consumption and destruction) and thrombomodulin expression (due to the action of TNFα and interleukin 1_β) (IL-1_β). This leads to a reduction in protein C activation (see Chapter 1). DIC may also be accompanied by an increase in plasminogen activator inhibitor-1 (PAI-1), leading to a reduction in fibrinolysis. These features will often by accompanied by thrombocytopenia (due to consumption of platelets in clot) and features of the causal disorder (see Table 8.15). Many of these altered biochemical parameters are sensitive to the presence of DIC, but are not very specific. In particular, fibrinogen is helpful when reduced, but may be maintained until late in the disease process. In such cases, serial measurements may be most helpful. At present, other tests – such as plasma levels of antithrombin, PAI-1, prothrombin fragment 1+2 (F1+2) and soluble fibrin levels – remain of research value only.

Out-with pregnancy, when there is evidence of a predisposing condition, a scoring system (using a combination of platelet count, fibrinogen, the prothrombin time, D-dimer or FDP) may be useful in the diagnosis of DIC. However, DIC may be more difficult to define in pregnancy, as D-dimer levels, FDP and fibrinogen all increase, and the APTT shortens even in normal pregnancy (see Chapter 1). Severe DIC may be obvious, but lesser forms will require reference to gestation-specific clotting factor ranges for diagnosis.

Treatment of DIC

The treatment, as in non-pregnant subjects, is directed to the cause of the DIC. Supportive therapy with coagulation factor products and platelets may be required if the patient is bleeding, or bleeding is likely. In amniotic fluid embolism, and in disorders such as acute promyelocytic leukemia, the predominant manifestation may be ischemia and thrombosis. In these circumstances, anticoagulation may be required. Occasionally, there is both bleeding and thrombosis, and a careful balancing act of therapeutic clotting factors (avoiding concentrated products where possible) and anticoagulation is required.

The coagulation and platelet product doses should be determined by frequent laboratory monitoring, with the aim of restoring platelets to at least $50 \times 10^9/l$ (perhaps even $80 \times 10^9/l$) and the coagulation screen to within reference limits, if the patient is bleeding. Traditionally, the fibrinogen is restored to $\geq 1 g/l$. Whether this is sufficient, given the higher reference range at the end of pregnancy, is unknown. Other therapies, such as heparin, antithrombin concentrate, or tissue factor pathway inhibitor do not yet have a proven role in the management of DIC. Recent evidence suggests that recombinant activated protein C therapy may have a beneficial effect on mortality from sepsis. However, a role for such therapy in DIC in pregnancy is untested.

Major obstetric hemorrhage

See Chapter 3.

Neonatal alloimmune thrombocytopenia (NAIT)

Although NAIT is not associated with maternal thrombocytopenia, it is a significant cause of neonatal thrombocytopenia, occurring in 1 in 1000–2000 live births. It can cause intracerebral hemorrhage (ICH), which most often occurs during or after delivery, although up to 10% of cases may occur prior to the onset of labor.

The disease is caused by transplacental passage of fetal platelets, which initiates a maternal reaction similar to that seen with red cells in RhD disease. This leads to the maternal production of antiplatelet antibodies directed at antigens on the fetal platelets (HPA inherited from the father). Five major HPA systems have been identified as causing NAIT. Although HPA-1a is the most commonly implicated antigen in the Caucasian population (>80% of cases), other HPA platelet glycoprotein antigens, such as HPA-5b (5–15% of cases), can also result in NAIT. In Asian populations, HPA-4a is commonly linked with the disorder.

Diagnosis of NAIT

The prevalence of the HPA-1a-negative platelet phenotype is about 2%. In most countries, there is no routine screening procedure for anti-HPA-1a, or anti-HPA-5b, so the first affected baby is usually diagnosed after birth. Ten per cent of ICH occur antepartum (often between 30 and 35 weeks gestation), and occasionally NAIT will be diagnosed in utero, when investigations have been carried out for other reasons. Sixty per cent of identified cases occur in first pregnancies that are otherwise uneventful, making it difficult to predict who may be at risk. The clinical presentation of the affected infant may vary from incidental thrombocytopenia and/or a purpura rash to the presence of ICH. NAIT can lead to developmental changes in 25% of affected subjects, with more severe disease resulting in motor dysfunction and intellectual impairment. The diagnosis may also come to light after investigations to exclude other causes of fetal thrombocytopenia, such as infection, birth defects, chromosomal abnormalities, intrauterine growth restriction (IUGR), hemangioma or a maternal thrombocytopenia. It may also be suspected where there has been a history of fetal ICH, recurrent miscarriage or fetal hydrocephalus. A diagnosis of NAIT should only be made after exclusion of maternal history of an autoimmune disorder, thrombocytopenia or drug abuse.

Predicting NAIT may be difficult, as antibody testing can produce conflicting results. A mother with a positive antibody test may have an unaffected infant and a mother with a negative result may have an affected infant. However, any woman with a history of severe disease, such as resulting in neonatal death, should be considered at risk and, consequently, tested for platelet alloimmunization. If platelet-specific antibodies are identified, antigen phenotyping of parental specimens is required to determine the platelet antigen system involved. Even in the absence of positive serology, parental antigen incompatibility can still be identified with antigen phenotyping. In general, parents should be assessed prior to a second pregnancy, so that the implicated antigen can be determined, and both diagnostic and management strategies can be discussed. If the father is heterozygous for the implicated antigen, it should be anticipated that the risk of recurrence, with the same parentage, will be 50%.

Investigations to determine the presence of a maternal alloantibody against a paternal platelet antigen should use a combination of sensitive techniques, as a maternal alloantibody may not be detectable in up to 20% of cases. In such cases, the diagnosis will have to rely upon the clinical history and the presence of a relevant HPA mismatch between the mother and father. When carrying out such investigations, it is important to exclude maternal platelet autoantibodies and HLA antibodies. In addition, the maternal and paternal platelet antigens should be determined, either by sensitive monoclonal antibody or genotyping techniques.

Treatment of NAIT

First pregnancy

As the platelet count may continue to fall in the first days after birth, infants should be monitored daily. The presence of significant thrombocytopenia requires ultrasound scanning for possible ICH. The passive thrombocytopenia from NAIT persists for 1–3 weeks postpartum, depending on the rate of removal of maternal platelet antibodies from the baby's circulation. Compatible HPA-1a negative or HPA-5b negative (as appropriate) allogenic platelets are most often used for the neonatal treatment. In some instances, washed, irradiated (to prevent graft versus host disease), maternal platelets may be used. If platelets are unavailable, high-dose Ig therapy, at a dose of 1g/day for 1–3 days, has been used. This requires 24–48 hours for an effect to be seen, but may be beneficial in up to 75% of cases.

Second pregnancy

Two potential strategies for the management of a second pregnancy are:

- the use of IVIgG ± steroids in the mother from around 24 weeks gestation to inhibit antibody production and reduce placental transfer;
- serial platelet transfusions for the fetus from around the same gestation.

At present, which management strategy is optimal is not yet clear. Indeed, a combination of these strategies may also be useful.

IVIgG has been reported to improve the fetal platelet count in only 27% of cases in some studies and in 66% in others, with an associated risk of ICH varying from 0 to 7%. Furthermore, IVIgG therapy requires monitoring of fetal blood count, which itself will require platelet cover. It has been suggested, however, that where the previous sibling was not severely affected, fetal platelet count monitoring may not be required.

The second strategy requires fetal full blood sampling from around 22–24 weeks gestation, with fetal platelet transfusions on a weekly basis into the intra-hepatic vein or placental cord. This has been associated with two fatalities in 12 managed pregnancies. Where the fetus is, or is suspected to be, affected, delivery will usually be by elective Cesarean section.

CHAPTER 9

Hereditary red cell disorders

Hemoglobinopathy

The hemoglobin molecule is a tetramer made up of two α-like globin chains and two β-like chains. The genes encoding the globin chains occur in two clusters on chromsomes 16 and 11. At different times in embryonic and fetal development the α-like chains can be either α or ζ-chains, and the β-like chains can be either β-, γ-, δ-, or ε-chains. This results in a mixture of embryonic, fetal and adult hemoglobins (Table 9.1). In late fetal development, the production of the fetal hemoglobin F (HbF) (α_2,γ_2) reduces, leaving a predominance of adult hemoglobin A (HbA) $(\alpha_2\beta_2)$ and <3.5% HbA$_2$ $(\alpha_2\delta_2)$.

Hemoglobin takes up oxygen at high oxygen saturation (in the lungs) and rapidly releases oxygen in the relatively hypoxic peripheral tissues. Changes in local pH, the red cell level of CO_2 and the red cell level of the compound 2,3-diphosphoglycerate (2,3-DPG) can all alter the affinity of hemoglobin for oxygen.

Hemoglobin's affinity for oxygen is also important to the developing fetus, as in general, HbF requires a higher affinity for oxygen than maternal HbA, to allow transfer of oxygen from the maternal circulation.

The group of disorders which result in the production of a defective hemoglobin are amongst the commonest maternal genetic disorders associated with an adverse pregnancy outcome. This group ranges from the thalassemias, which are characterized by a failure of production of a hemoglobin chain, to genetic

Table 9.1 – Hemoglobin (Hb) development

Stage	Name	α-chain type	β-chain type	Hb combination
Embryo	Hb Gower 1	ζ	ε	$\zeta_2\varepsilon_2$
	Hb Portland	ζ	γ	$\zeta_2\gamma_2$
	Hb Gower 2	α	ε	$\alpha_2\varepsilon_2$
Fetal	HbF	α	γ	$\alpha_2\gamma_2$
Adult	HbA	α	β	$\alpha_2\beta_2$
	Hb A$_2$	α	δ	$\alpha_2\delta_2$

changes that result in an alteration of the conformational structure of the hemoglobin (Table 9.2). Such conformational change can result in an alteration in oxygen affinity, or an increased susceptibility of the hemoglobin molecule to hypoxic damage. Principal amongst these are those disorders in which hypoxia leads to the formation of a rigid hemoglobin structure: the sickling disorders.

The management of pregnancy in subjects known, or suspected, to have such disorders can be divided into the management of an affected mother, the assessment of the risks of fetal transmission from a maternal carrier and the management of an affected fetus.

The thalassemias

The thalassemias are a heterogeneous group of genetic disorders of hemoglobin synthesis: they are named after the hemoglobin that is deficient and can be described as shown in Table 9.2. The mutation may result in a reduced rate of production from the affected gene (for the β gene the notation used for this is 'β^+' and for the α gene the notation is 'α^+'), or result in no globin chain synthesis at all (again for the β gene the notation for this is 'β^0' and for the α gene the notation is 'α^0'). The majority of thalassemias are inherited in a Mendelian recessive manner and there are known mutations that affect hemoglobin transcription, mRNA processing, translation and post-translational modification.

Table 9.2 – Hemoglobinopathy types

Hemoglobinopathy type	Subtypes
α	Deletional Non-deletional
β	Deletional Non-deletional Normal HbA_2 variant Dominant variant
$\delta\beta$	Deletional Non-deletional
γ	–
δ	Deletional Non-deletional
$\epsilon\gamma\delta\beta$	Large β gene deletion
Hereditary persistance of HbF (HPFH)	Deletional Non-deletional

Table 9.3 – Types of thalassemia intermedia

Beta thalassemias	Homozygous mild beta thalassemia
	Mild compound beta heterozygote
	Dominant beta thalassemia trait
	Compound heterozygote of beta and a beta variant (Hb C, E, Lepore, $\delta\beta$)
Alpha and beta combinations	β^+ with HbH disease
	β^+ with α^+ or α^0 mutations
	Heterozygote β, co-inheritance of an extra α ($\alpha\alpha\alpha$)
Beta mutations with increased γ-chains	Homozygous β thalassemia with HPFH
	Homozygous β thalassemia, with a γ promoter mutation

Given the diversity of genetic defects, and the possibility of genetic combinations, thalassemias (irrespective of their molecular basis) are often classified by their clinical effects into thalassemia minor, thalassemia intermedia and thalassemia major. In general, thalassemia carriers are often symptomless and fall into the minor category. Intermediate levels are more severely affected and may often have anemia, although this does not require regular transfusion (Table 9.3). In its major form, thalassemia presents with a lifelong transfusion dependency.

Alpha thalassemia

The α globin chain is common to both HbF and HbA, and deficiencies in the gene (the alpha thalassemias), are found in subjects of Middle Eastern, Mediterranean or African descent. As noted above, the human α globin gene cluster is located on chromosome 16 and, normally, each individual has a total of four α globin genes, with two on each chromosome. Although these genes are identical, the α-2 globin gene location contributes significantly more α-globin chain production to hemoglobin than the α-1 gene location. There are gene mutations that can affect either one, or both, of the α globin genes on each chromosome. Alpha thalassemia most often results from a deletion of these genes, although non-deletional forms also occur (Table 9.4). The severity of the thalassemia phe-

Table 9.4 – Mechanism of alpha thalassemia

Hb Barts hydrops fetalis results from severe '(--/--)'
HbH commonly results from severe '(--/--α)'
Hb Bart and HbH have $\uparrow$ O$_2$ affinity $\rightarrow$ poor oxygen delivery
Hb Bart and HbH precipitate $\rightarrow$ hemolysis

notype depends on the effect of the mutation on the production of α globin chains (either complete deletion or reduced production) and the contribution of the affected gene to the overall hemoglobin production.

The four genes are described as '($\alpha\alpha,\alpha\alpha$)' in a normal individual, with a '-' used to describe a mutation. Mutations can then result in a number of combinations. A single gene mutation is described as '(α-,$\alpha\alpha$)'. A two-gene mutation is described as '(α-,α-)' if one mutation is found on each chromosome and '($\alpha\alpha$,--)' if both mutations are found on the same chromosome. If three mutations occur, this is represented as '(--,-α)'. Finally, if there are four mutations then this is described as '(--,--)'. In addition, and as noted above, mutations which lead to no gene output are also described as an 'α^0', mutation and mutations which result in some gene production are described as an 'α^+' mutation.

In general, one- and two-gene mutations produce a symptomless carrier state, but two mutations on the same chromosome, i.e. '(-,$\alpha\alpha$)', produce a more severe hematology pattern than when one mutation occurs on one chromosome and one on the other, i.e. '(α-,α-)'.

When both the mother and father are carriers of an 'α^0' '(--,$\alpha\alpha$)', mutation, then there are four possible outcomes:

- The fetus is normal, i.e. '($\alpha\alpha,\alpha\alpha$)';
- The fetus carries the paternal mutation, i.e. '(--,$\alpha\alpha$)';
- The fetus carries the maternal mutation, i.e. '(--,$\alpha\alpha$)'; or
- The fetus inherits the 'α^0' mutation from both parents and is therefore '(--,--)'.

In 'α^0' mutations, when there is no α-chain production, the fetus attempts to form tetramers of the available β-chain (γ), forming a γ-tetramer that is called Hb Barts. Hb Barts has a high oxygen affinity and, if it is major hemoglobin, leads to a severe anemia during fetal development, with the risk of cardiac failure. This most often leads to stillbirth, or neonatal death in the third trimester (called Hb Barts hydrops fetalis); the name comes from St Bartholomew's Hospital in London, where the condition was first described in a baby of Chinese origin.

Where an 'α^0' carrier with '(--,$\alpha\alpha$)' is partnered by an 'α^+' carrier with '(α-,$\alpha\alpha$)', this also results in four possible outcomes:

- The fetus is normal, i.e. '($\alpha\alpha,\alpha\alpha$)';
- The fetus carries the 'α^+' mutation, i.e. '(α-,$\alpha\alpha$)';
- The fetus carries the 'α^0' mutation, i.e. '(--,$\alpha\alpha$)'; or
- The fetus inherits both the 'α^+' and 'α^0' mutations, i.e. '(--/-α)'.

In such circumstances, unlike Hb Barts hydrops fetalis, as there is some α-chain production, the fetus is able to form some $\alpha\beta$ hemoglobin, but also attempts to form a tetramer of the available β-chains. This results in the formation of some β-chain tetramers and results in HbH disease. These HbH (β-chain) tetramers can be seen in the cell and are called HbH inclusions. The abnormal β-chain tetramers also result in a hemoglobin with a high oxygen affinity. Such hemoglobins fail to deliver adequate oxygen to the tissues and these tetramers also tend to precipitate within red cells, which shortens red cell survival by hemolysis in the spleen (see Table 9.4).

Alpha thalassemia: problems in pregnancy
The problems in pregnancy can be considered from the viewpoint of maternal carriers of one- or two-gene mutations, maternal carriers with an affected fetus, the problems associated with maternal carriage of HbH disease and the features of a fetus with Hb Barts.

Maternal alpha thalassemia carriers
As noted above, women with one or two 'α^0' gene deletions,'$(\alpha\text{-},\alpha\alpha)$', '$\alpha\text{-},\alpha\text{-}$)' or '$(-\ -,\alpha\alpha)$', are usually symptom-free and have a normal pregnancy outcome. Despite the fact that she is usually symptom-free, if a mother is carrying a fetus affected by Hb Barts, she has a higher risk of pregnancy complications as a consequence of placentomegaly. It has been estimated that at least 50% of subjects carrying an Hb Barts fetus will have evidence of pregnancy-induced hypertension and around 30% will have evidence of pre-eclampsia. It may be that other complications, such as polyhydramnios, antepartum and postpartum hemorrhage, disseminated intravascular coagulation (DIC), placental abruption, premature labor and malpresentation, are also more common in such women (Table 9.5).

A mother with HbH disease
The majority of subjects are diagnosed in childhood, perhaps coming to light as a result of acute hemolysis induced by infection (when hemoglobin levels may fall by up to 3g/dl). The clinical features of an adult with HbH disease vary from mild asymptomatic anemia (commonly with a hemoglobin of >8g/dl) to a severe trans-

Table 9.5 – Features of Hb Barts hydrops fetalis

Fetal
Third trimester stillbirth/neonatal death
Large placental volume
Pallor
Generalized edema
Marked hepatosplenomegaly
Other congenital anomalies
Hb 6–8g/dl
80% Hb Barts/20% Hb Portland
Maternal
Pre-eclampsia (PET)
APH and PPH due to placentomegaly

APH, Antepartum hemorrhage; PPH, Postpartum hemorrhage

fusion-dependent anemia, with jaundice, hepatosplenomegaly, growth restriction and bone abnormalities. The symptoms of maternal HbH disease are variable, with mild to moderate hemolysis being the predominant feature. The level of HbH inclusions may be increased by pyrexial illness. Iron overload, even in the absence of previous transfusion, is not uncommon in subjects from Far Eastern countries. In addition, gallstones are not infrequent, and 20–70% of cases will have hepatomegaly or splenomegaly. Infections, fever, oxidative drugs, parvovirus infection, as well as pregnancy itself, may worsen the anemia (Table 9.6).

Fetal alpha thalssemia carriers

In newborn infants with '(-α/-α)', a variable quantity of Hb Barts (0.5–2%) is detectable at birth. In cases of '(– –/αα)' carriage, Hb Barts may constitute up to 10% of the hemoglobin at delivery, although this disappears by 6 months of age, as there are sufficient α-chains for hemoglobin synthesis. Fetal carriers of mild α-chain mutations are, as adults, unlikely to be affected during development, but occasional HbH inclusions may be detected in the blood.

Fetal HbH disease

The more severe HbH disease, '(– –/-α)', most often presents in childhood as a mild to moderate hemolytic anemia, although fetal HbH hydrops has rarely been reported in the literature. There have also been isolated case reports of an association between HbH disease and skeletal changes, facial dysmorphia and retinopathy.

Fetal Hb Barts hydrops fetalis

In South East Asia, 'α^0' mutations are common, and are the commonest cause of hydrops fetalis in that region, where they may account for 1 in 4 perinatal deaths. Hb Barts hydrops fetalis has also been reported in subjects of Mediterranean descent.

In Hb Barts hydrops fetalis, γ-tetramers lead to hemoglobin instability, severe anemia and extramedullary hemopoiesis (leading to hepatosplenomegaly). As

Table 9.6 – Clinical features of HbH disease

Survival to adulthood
Inheritance of '(--,-α)' or homozygous non-deletion 'α⁺α⁺'
Variable anemia
Variable splenomegaly
Periodic hemolysis with oxidant drugs or infection
Prominent red cell HbH inclusions
Hb 7–10g/dl
<40% HbH, variable HbA and HbA_2

the change from ζ-chains to α-chains occurs by the 7th week of gestation, there is a lack of fetal oxygenation from early in development. This results in fetal hypoxia, abnormal organogenesis and placental enlargement. A number of congenital anomalies have also been reported in association with Hb Barts, which include abnormal brain, cardiac, skeletal or urinary tract development.

The clinical signs on Hb Barts-delivered fetus may vary from signs of cardiac failure to gross edema, hepatosplenomegaly and pallor (see Table 9.5). Although the vast majority of fetuses with Hb Barts hydrops fetalis die, there are a number of cases of severe alpha thalassemia which survive, to be maintained on transfusion and chelation regimes, with or without, the use of subsequent bone marrow transplantation.

Alpha thalassemia: diagnosis in pregnancy
Diagnosis of maternal carriers
Carriage of alpha thalassemia is associated with a mean red cell volume (MCV) <80fl (often <70fl) with a mean red cell hemoglobin (MCH) <27pg, with, very often, no evidence of anemia (Figure 9.1). In such cases, if iron deficiency is excluded, then carriage of thalassemia should be suspected. If suspected in one parent, the other parent should be examined to exclude a hypochromic/microcytic blood picture. There should always be a high index of suspicion if there is a previous family history of hydrops fetalis.

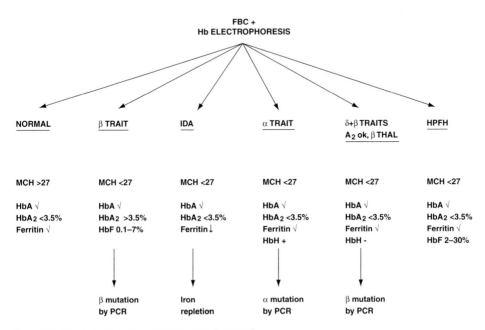

Figure 9.1 Discrimination of hypochromia and microcytosis
FBC, Full blood count; Hb, Hemoglobin; HPFH, Hereditary persistence of HbF; IDA, Iron deficiency anemia; MCH, Mean red cell hemoglobin; PCR, Polymerase chain reaction; Thal, Thalassemia.

Confirmation of carriage of alpha thalassemia trait requires a number of additional investigations. The search for HbH inclusions in the blood film is often included in the screening for alpha thalassemia, although this can be problematic given the infrequency of these inclusions in minor carrier states. A raised level of HbA_2 (>3.5%) in someone with hypochromia and microcytosis often suggests carriage of a beta rather than alpha thalassemia. The presence of a normal level of HbA_2 in such individuals points towards alpha thalassemia carriage. A normal level can occur, however, if the subject is a carrier of both alpha and beta thalassemia traits. Carriers of some alpha thalassemia mutations, such as '-SEA' may have detectable levels of ζ globin chains in red cells that can be detected by immunophenotyping, although larger mutations may result in no detectable ζ-chains. Although the diagnosis of alpha thalassemia is often made on the basis of the absence of iron deficiency and/or other hemoglobinopathy in someone with a hypochromic anemia (with or without HbH inclusions), for counseling it is necessary to determine the exact parental mutation. This can be achieved by a polymerase chain reaction (PCR) technique or Southern blot analysis.

Diagnosis of Hb Barts hydrops fetalis

In a case of suspected Hb Barts hydrops fetalis, ultrasonography may detect placentomegaly as early as 10 weeks gestation, and hydropic changes in the fetus are often evident at <20 weeks gestation. Fetal tissue (obtained by chorionic villus sampling (CVS) in the first trimester or by amniocentesis in the second) can be examined by PCR or Southern blot analysis for an alpha thalassemia mutation. As with all such fetal sampling, contamination with maternal DNA, or difficulties in establishing paternity, can be problematic. Examination of the fetal blood by cordocentesis in the second trimester will also permit examination of the expressed fetal hemoglobins by hemoglobin electrophoresis. A normal second trimester fetus will have predominantly HbF and ≤10% HbA, but in a fetus with Hb Barts the predominant hemoglobin will be Hb Barts (γ_4), with <20% Hb Portland and possibly some HbH (β_4).

Diagnosis of fetal carriage of alpha thalassemia traits

The detection of less severely affected infants, with either carriage of an α^0 '$(--,\alpha\alpha)$' mutation, or HbH disease, can be achieved by detection of HbH or Hb Barts in neonatal samples. Such detection may also indicate those parents at risk of a future affected child.

Alpha thalassemia: treatment in pregnancy

The carriage of minor thalassemic traits is unlikely to require specific intervention in pregnancy other than attendance to folic acid supplements and the exclusion of fetal carriage of severe thalassemia.

In maternal HbH disease, pre-existing anemia will be exacerbated by the physiological hemodilution associated with pregnancy (Table 9.7). Consequently, all mothers should attend to folic acid supplementation, as folate deficiency often

Table 9.7 – Maternal HbH treatment in pregnancy

Folic acid
Avoid antioxidant drugs
If Hb <6g/dl consider transfusion
Treatment of pre-eclampsia (PET) and gallstones
Screening for infant carriage of thalassemia

accompanies chronic hemolysis. Antioxidant drugs should be avoided. From the limited literature it appears that, in general, maternal HbH disease is consistent with a normal pregnancy outcome. In carriers there is, of course, the potential for transmission of either the '(– –)' or the '(- α)' mutation to the fetus (see above). If the hemoglobin falls to <6g/dl, there may be a case to transfuse the mother to improve maternal and fetal oxygenation. There are some reports that pre-eclampsia may be more common in mothers who have HbH disease. At present, however, the role of maternal HbH disease in other pregnancy problems, such as miscarriage and cardiac failure, requires further study.

Beta thalassemia

The beta thalassemias are found in those of Baltic, Mediterranean, Middle Eastern, African, Indian, Southern Chinese and South-East Asian extraction. Akin to the situation in alpha thalassemia, the defect of β-chains in beta thalassemia leads to the formation of α-chain tetramers, which interfere with the maturation of the red cell and result in red cell destruction within the marrow and the spleen (Table 9.8). In beta thalassemia, this reduction in β-chains is accompanied by an increase in δ-chain hemoglobin production, which is identified as an increase in the level of HbA_2 $(\alpha_2\delta_2)$.

In the homozygous, or compound heterozygous, beta thalassemic states, there is a lifelong chronic dyserythropoietic anemia, which results in splenomegaly and

Table 9.8 – Mechanism of beta thalassemia

α tetramers $\rightarrow$ hemolysis in bone marrow and spleen
Reduced α-chains, or increased HbF improves symptoms
$\uparrow$ HbA_2 is common

Beta thalassemia major presents in the first year
Insufficient transfusion $\rightarrow$ deformity and infection
Insufficient chelation $\rightarrow$ iron overload

skeletal deformity. This clinical picture is ameliorated by any mutation that reduces the amount of α-chain production, as this reduces the imbalance in the relative amounts of α- and β-chains, and reduces dyserythropoiesis. The disease is also ameliorated in subjects who have also inherited hereditary persistence of HbF (HPFH).

Subjects affected by severe beta thalassemia usually present within the first year of life, with symptoms of anemia and evidence of splenomegaly. The progression of the disease is heavily dependent upon the adequacy of transfusion and iron chelation. In the absence of adequate transfusion there may be profound anemia, marked skeletal deformity of the long bones and skull, recurrent infections, and death within the first few years. With adequate transfusion there may be few symptoms and no development of a hyperdynamic state. By the second decade, however, the effect of transfusion-related iron overload will result in adrenal, pancreatic, hepatic and cardiac failure (Table 9.9). This may also compromise sexual development and, in the absence of adequate chelation, death is often due to cardiac failure or dysrythmia. With a new generation who have received adequate and safe transfusion, and adequate chelation, there is the hope of an improved life expectancy.

Beta thalassemia: problems in pregnancy
As with alpha thalassemia, carriers of beta thalassemia are usually symptom-free, although a mild anemia may develop in pregnancy. More significant anemias may occur in relation to dietary deficiency. In such cases there may be a requirement for folate and iron supplementation.

As noted above, females with homozygous beta thalassemia usually suffer from endocrine abnormalities due to iron overload. This results in a failure of pubertal growth and severely delayed sexual development, and hypogonadotrophic hypogonadism. On account of this, only a small number of successful pregnancies are reported in the literature. Some of these have occurred spontaneously and others have required stimulation of ovulation.

In severely affected individuals, a number of risks have to be considered before embarking on pregnancy. These include the cardiovascular risk to the mother and the impact of other iron-overload effects, such as diabetes mellitus and hypothyroidism, that may be present. Cardiac complications are associated

Table 9.9 – Iron overload in beta thalassemia

Iron overload is evident in the second decade
Pituitary iron overload → impaired sexual development
Hepatic iron overload → cirrhosis
Cardiac iron overload → dysrythmia and failure
Endocrine overload → hypothyroidism and diabetes mellitus

with mortality in both transfused and un-transfused patients, which is important in pregnancy where major changes in cardiac function occur, with a substantial increase in cardiac output evident by 12 weeks gestation that may be compounded by anemia.

Serum ferritin may provide a reasonable reflection of hepatic iron stores, but does not relate well to pituitary or cardiac deposition. Myocardial iron deposition can provoke left ventricular dysfunction, along with superimposed myocarditis. Where significant left ventricular dysfunction is present, or when significant arrthymias have occurred, then pregnancy may be best avoided. Most non-invasive cardiac imaging techniques are relatively insensitive for detecting early cardiac iron deposition. However, magnetic resonance imaging (MRI) techniques can now quantify cardiac iron deposition and relate these to left ventricular dimensions.

The most common adverse event reported in successful pregnancies is the need for Cesarean section, given that there is a high risk of cephalopelvic disproportion. This is due to the small stature of the mother when the unaffected fetus exhibits normal growth. The risk of pregnancy-related thrombosis in those women who have previously undergone splenectomy is unknown, but there is a risk of mechanical difficulties from an enlarged spleen if it is still present. In those mothers who have undergone splenectomy, the need for antibiotic prophylaxis and vaccination should be remembered, as well as the need for thrombo-prophylaxis (see Chapter 8, Table 8.10).

In mothers with well-treated (hemoglobin chronically maintained >10g/dl) and well-chelated beta thalassemia, or in women with thalassemia intermedia (with no evidence of bone abnormality and a hemoglobin level >7g/dl without regular transfusion), there is a reasonable pregnancy success rate. In one study of women who had undergone regular transfusion and chelation, and had normal left ventricular function with no evidence of a red cell autoantibody at conception, a successful pregnancy was achieved in 21 of 23 pregnancies. In this study, one miscarriage and one fatal fetal abnormality (perhaps related to maternal iron overload) was reported. All mothers had their chelation stopped at least by the confirmation of conception. Two mothers suffered biliary colic due to gallstones, but there was no evidence of significant cardiac, renal, hepatic or endocrine deterioration in any of the subjects, and the fetal outcome was comparable to that of the general population. This suggests that a careful pre-pregnancy medical assessment may result in appropriate counseling and the possibility of a successful pregnancy in at least some women with beta thalassemia major.

Beta thalassemia: diagnosis in pregnancy
Maternal
In beta thalassemia carriers, the full blood count reveals a reduction in the MCV and MCH. Hemoglobin electrophoresis reveals the presence of normal HbA, with elevated levels of HbA_2 (4–6%), and perhaps an elevated level of HbF.

In homozygous, or compound heterozygous, beta thalassemia major, HbA ($\alpha_2\beta_2$) is absent and only HbF and HbA$_2$ are evident. In less severe (β^+) thalassemia, HbF may constitute <90% of the hemoglobin. As the measured HbA$_2$ level is an average of all cells, this may well be within normal limits. As with alpha thalassemia, DNA analysis is needed for prenatal diagnosis.

Fetal

At birth, absence of HbA is a feature of beta thalassemia major. Although there is little evidence that early detection is cost or clinically effective, early detection will allow the commencement of surveillance and the early onset of transfusion therapy. When heel stab cards are used for diagnosis, storage changes may occur if there is a long delay in the analysis of the neonatal sample, making identification of hemoglobins difficult. If a cord sample is used for neonatal diagnosis, cross-contamination with maternal blood may be a problem. This can be suspected if there is a high level of HbA, but careful cleaning of the cord may markedly reduce the risk of such contamination. Hemoglobin identification can be achieved by cellulose acetate electrophoresis, although immuno-electrophoresis and high-performance liquid chromatography (HPLC) are more sensitive methods. The nature of the genetic mutation can be determined by a number of different PCR-based techniques, often using a combination of probes that relate to mutations that are common in the ethnic population of the patient under study. The exact screening technique used depends upon the ethnic mix and knowledge of predominant mutations.

Beta thalassemia major: treatment in pregnancy

Transfusion requirements increase with increasing gestation, and the aim should be to maintain the hemoglobin concentration >10g/dl. When transfusion is insufficient there is the risk of fetal hypoxia and pre-term delivery. As in the non-pregnant, such blood should be screened for hepatitis A, B and C, and HIV, and the cytomegalovirus (CMV) status of the individuals should also be taken into account. All individuals undergoing regular transfusion programs should be vaccinated against hepatitis B and A. They should also have a red cell phenotype determined prior to the onset of such transfusion programs (see Chapter 2) so that, whenever possible, blood is used that is compatible with this phenotype to prevent red cell alloimmunization. In the UK, blood is routinely leukodepleted, but if this is not the case, consideration should be given to bedside leukocyte filtration to reduce the risk of febrile non-hemolytic transfusion reactions as well as CMV transmission. In such individuals there may also be a role for cell salvage at delivery.

There is evidence, from animal studies, that the chelating agent desferrioxamine may be teratogenic (Table 9.10). Also, as the newer chelating agents have no safety track record in pregnancy, the role of continuing chelation therapy during pregnancy is not yet defined. The increase in serum ferritin in such subjects is likely to be <10% over the course of pregnancy. However, whether this represents a reduction in iron loading from hemodilution or fetal usage of iron requires further study. Currently, in the vast majority of planned pregnancies, chelating agents will be stopped when conception is confirmed, but may be restarted after delivery, even if breastfeeding. There is also a suggestion that vitamin C therapy should be stopped in pregnancy, as it may increase intestinal absorption of iron. Folic acid, at a dose of at least 5mg should be utilized in all subjects as the chronic hemolytic state may result in folate deficiency, with the attendant risks upon the maternal blood as well as fetal neural tube development. The mother will require additional monitoring if there is evidence of significant maternal endocrine dysfunction, particularly for thyroid and parathyroid dysfunction and glucose intolerance. At term, consideration should be given to the possibility of cephalopelvic disproportion (see above) when planning delivery. In those women with hypersplenism, thrombocytopenia ($<80 \times 10^9/l$) may contraindicate neuraxial anesthesia. The presence of short stature, spinal abnormalities and osteoporosis (and possible vertebral collapse), and disturbed linear growth associated with spinal cartilaginous dysplasia due to childhood chelation therapy, should also be taken into consideration with neuraxial anesthesia. Ideally, pre-pregnancy spinal X–ray examination should be performed in women with these complications.

Thalassemia intermedia

This term covers a variety of thalassemic disorders, in which a combination of defects results in an anemia that is more severe than that found in carrier states but does not result in lifelong transfusion dependence (see Table 9.3). This clinical definition includes HbC or HbE thalassemia, Hb Lepore and thalassemic syndromes that arise as a result of a variety of combinations of α, β and $\delta\beta$ deficiencies. As noted above, the inheritance of an α-chain mutation, along with a homozygous β-chain disorder, will ameliorate the clinical picture by reducing the β/α-chain imbalance and the consequent ineffective erythropoiesis.

Table 9.10 – Management of beta thalassemia in pregnancy

Pre-pregnancy assessment if possible
Assess cardiac/endocrine reserve
Beta thalassemia carriers at risk of a mild anemia in pregnancy
Continue folic acid throughout pregnancy
Stop vitamin C
?Stop chelation
Consider infection risk if previous splenectomy
Consider risk of cephalopelvic disproportion

These combinations result in clinical syndromes which run from mild anemia to the more obvious signs of a chronic hemolytic anemia, such as folate deficiency, gallstones, leg ulceration, infection and extramedullary hemopoiesis (with skeletal abnormality and splenomegaly).

Stem cell transplantation

It is now possible to treat the major hemoglobinopathies with hematopoietic stem cell transplantation from a human leukocyte antigen – (HLA)-compatible donor, and there is now a considerable body of literature reporting successful treatment of thalassemia major, as well as, sickle-cell disorders.

Transplant procedures are not, however, an easy option, as they require, at present, intensive chemotherapy to ablate the existing bone marrow. Such a procedure also necessitates a period of profound neutropenia and thrombocytopenia. This carries a significant procedure-related morbidity and mortality, and the transplant also requires subsequent lifelong immunosuppression. There are also the long-term problems of graft versus host disease and, in children, growth disturbance (particularly after radiotherapy marrow conditioning). Such procedures also carry a greater risk in older subjects, in those with iron overload and in those with viral infections of the liver. Furthermore, a graft failure rate of around 10% has been reported in the transplantation of sickle-cell disorders.

At present, such procedures are therefore limited to younger, severely affected individuals, where there is a suitable donor – preferably a sibling, as this carries a lower risk of graft versus host disease and, in general, less procedural mortality than an unrelated transplant – and where there is little evidence of iron overload or organ failure. In developed countries, however, <30% of indivudals have a suitable family donor and, indeed, such transplants are only pertinent to countries where there are the considerable resources and facilities required for a successful outcome.

A number of developments may increase the applicability of hematopoietic stem cell transplantation for thalassemia and sickling disorders in the future. The growth of bone marrow registries and cord stem cell banks will increase the availability of suitable donors, although, at present, the role for unrelated allogenic transplants in hemoglobinopathies is not yet defined. As noted in Chapter 2, cord stem cells may also offer the additional benefit of less stringent matching requirements. It has also been reported that a number of transplants for thalassemia have resulted in the formation of a stable chimer of donor and recipient in the marrow. This appears to lead to a reduction in the severity of graft versus host disease, whilst maintaining a useful amelioration of thalassemic symptoms. This is one of the rationales for a reduction in the intensity of the bone marrow conditioning regimens in thalassemia transplants from that required for transplantation in malignant conditions. Indeed, successful transplants for hemoglobinopathies have been reported with purine analog conditioning, although a reduction in the dose of cyclophsophamide used is associated with an increase in graft rejection and graft failure. On account of this, when a transplant is being considered for a young, otherwise fit, individual with a likelihood of a good outcome, then full conditioning is probably to be recommended. Lesser induction regimens may be considered for the older, less fit, individual.

Sickle-cell disease

Sickle-cell disease is the most common hemoglobinopathy in the USA, with around 8% of African Americans carrying the sickle-cell gene. Disorders which result in clinically significant sickling of the red cell result from the combination of a sickle-cell gene on one β-chain combined with (on the other chromosome) either:

■ Another sickle-cell mutation (HbSS); or

■ An HbC mutation (HbSC); or

■ A beta thalassemia gene (HbSβ⁰).

Sickle-cell disease can result in a lifelong crippling hemolytic disorder (characterized by crises caused by infection, aplasia, infarction and hemolysis) to a diagnosis only detected on a routine blood film examination (Table 9.11). This variation in symptoms can be due to the co-inheritance of other hemoglobin changes, such as the HPFH or α thalassemia. The overall clinical expression of the disease is also highly dependent on the availability of health care.

Table 9.11 – Sickle-cell disease features

Major sickling occurs in	SS, Sβ⁰, SC, SD disease
Crisis management	Hemolytic Aplastic Infarction: pain, bones, cerebral ischemia of arterial origin (CIAO), myocardial infarction Sequestration – liver, spleen (children), lung
Symptom amelioration	Influence of ↑ HbF Treatment with hydroxybutyrate (↑ HbF) Influence of healthcare
Transfusion management	Alloimmunization Iron overload Blood-borne infections
Infection risk	Osteomyelitis Capsulated organisms
Fetal risks of maternal sickle-cell disease	Intrauterine growth restriction (IUGR) Pre-term delivery

Sickle-cell disease most often presents with infarction of the fingers in childhood, called dactylitis. There may be also recurrent infection or sequestration of blood into the spleen causing profound anemia. However, due to repeated infarction, it is unusual for there to be a palpable spleen by the teenage years, and indeed there is, more often, hematological evidence of hyposplenism. These infarction crises are often precipitated by dehydration or infection, and present with pain which can be localized or diffuse. Childhood infection with any organism, but particularly parvovirus, may trigger an aplastic crisis with profound anemia. In childhood, infarction crises may also present with a cerebral ischemia of arterial origin (CIAO). There is also the possibility of sequestration of sickle cells into the liver, spleen and lungs. Such lung sequestration will result in a rapid deterioration in oxygenation and is a common cause of death.

With repeated crises there may be the development of bone deformity, osteomyelitis, renal failure, myocardial infarction, leg ulceration, gallstones and cardiac failure. Indeed, almost 30% of young adults with sickle-cell disease develop a widespread vasculopathy with glomerulosclerosis, retinopathy, restrictive lung disease and stroke. With repeated transfusions there may also be an increased risk of blood-borne infections and iron overload.

In SS disease, but more severely in the case of SC disease, there is an increased risk of a proliferation of blood vessels in the retina (due to hypoxia), ultimately causing vitreous hemorrhage, retinal detachment and blindness. This lifelong series of painful crises and hospital admission also results in a disturbance of schooling and development.

Sickle-cell disease in pregnancy

It is very likely that maternal carriage of a sickle-cell trait is associated with an uncomplicated maternal and fetal outcome. In such individuals, sickling only occurs at PaO_2 levels <15mmHg and is very unlikely to give rise to clinical problems in normal obstetric practice.

As noted above, the outcome of pregnancy in mothers with sickling disorders is heavily dependent upon the adequacy of maternal health care. In the USA, a maternal mortality rate is likely to be of the order of 0.25–0.5%, with some 99% of pregnancies (which were viable after 28 weeks) resulting in a live birth. Although the majority of pregnancies result in a healthy child, around half of pregnancies are complicated by at least one painful crisis, and SS patients are more likely to require hospital admissions. It is possible, however, that these painful crises are no more frequent than would be expected in the same women when not pregnant, and the rate of pyelonephritis has been reported to be no greater than in women without a sickling disorder in some, but not all, studies.

There is likely to be an increased risk of pre-eclampsia, which has been reported to occur in 14% of subjects with a sickling disorders, including those with only a sickle-cell trait. There is also an effect on fetal growth, with 70–85% of pregnancies resulting in a baby below the 50th centile for the population and, in up to 27%, the baby is below the 10th centile. This may relate to the known association of sickling disorders and placental infarction, although the risk of a small baby has also been linked with the occurrence of anemic events during pregnancy and inversely related to maternal HbF levels.

Anemic events do not appear to be limited to any specific gestation, but they are more common in sickle/thalassemia combinations than they are in pure sickle-cell disease (Table 9.12). In African Americans, the incidence of acute chest syndrome appears not to be increased in pregnancy. There is, however, likely to be an increased risk of premature rupture of membranes, pre-term delivery and postpartum maternal infection. Multiple pregnancies, as a result of a reduction in available nutrition and oxygen transfer to the fetus, appear to be at more risk of poor fetal growth. Whether the use of narcotic analgesia affects fetal development is not clear, although some may have a vasoconstrictive effect on the placental vasculature.

An increased risk of a growth-restricted baby and postpartum infection has also been reported in subjects with SC disease, although there is a lesser need for transfusion and fewer painful crises in SC than in SS disease. In developing countries the outcome of pregnancy in subjects with a major sickling disorder may be substantially worse, with maternal mortality approaching 25% and a fetal mortality approaching 40%.

Sickle-cell disorders: diagnosis in pregnancy

Sickle-cell trait results in no change to the hematological indices, i.e. the MCV and MCH are normal unless another hemogloibin disorder is present. The trait is diagnosed by a positive sickle test and the demonstration of both an HbA and HbS band on gel electrophoresis, indicating the presence of both normal and sickle hemoglobin.

Sickle-cell disease is diagnosed by the presence of anemia, sickled red cells on the blood film, blood film appearances of hyposplenism, a positive sickle test: it is confirmed by the hemoglobin electrophoresis pattern of HbS, and elevated HbF with no HbA. The presence of a microcytosis may suggest the co-inheritance of thalassemia, or the presence of iron deficiency. A higher than expected hemo-

Table 9.12 – Causes of anemia in sickle-cell disease in pregnancy

Blood loss
Infection
Vitamin deficiency
Aplastic crisis
Inflammation

globin level (11–13g/dl) may indicate the presence of HbC, or co-inheritance of another hemoglobin variant.

To determine the presence of sickle-cell disease in the fetus, the father (where paternity can be assured) should be screened for the presence of any hemoglobinopathy. The presence of sickle-cell disease in the fetus can be confirmed by the analysis of fetal DNA for sickle-cell mutations using techniques outlined previously (see Chapter 4). The newborn is protected from sickling in the first few months of life due to the high level of HbF at birth.

Sickle-cell disease: treatment in pregnancy

General management
In all subjects with a major sickling disorder, treatment must include the prevention of infection. This is achieved with prophylactic penicillin and the use of pneumococcal, meningococcal and *Hemophilus influenzae* vaccinations, with antimalarial prophylaxis where appropriate (Table 9.13). The management of a painful crisis involves adequate pain control (with opiates if required), treatment of any infection, and maintenance of oxygenation and hydration.

A worsening of anemia may be precipitated by a number of events (see Table 9.12). In general, regular blood transfusion is not required. If, however, there is evidence of a falling hemoglobin level (indicating an increase in hemolysis), and especially if there is evidence of a falling reticulocyte count (indicating an impending aplastic phase), then transfusion should be given. When transfusion is required and the hemoglobin level is already <5g/dl, it may be that a top-up transfusion to 12–14g/dl will result in sufficient dilution of the sickle cells (to reduce sickling) to the desired target level of <30% of the circulating red cells. When transfusion is required at a higher hemoglobin level (8–10g/dl), then a partial exchange transfusion should be carried out (removing 500ml by phlebotomy whilst transfusing 2 red cell units).

Lung and sequestration crises require close monitoring. Sequestration into the lung may present with fever, cough, pleuritic chest pain and evidence of lung infiltrates on X-ray. In such cases, the patient is likely to require intensive-care therapy with oxygen support, monitoring, hydration and exchange transfusion. In the ill patient with a major sickling disorder, the possibility of sequestration into liver or spleen may be assessed by regular measurement of the hemoglobin level and assessment of the liver and spleen size. If acute sequestration occurs, the hemoglobin level can drop within hours and urgent transfusion will be required.

It is recommended that a subject with a recent episode of CIAO should receive regular red cell transfusions to keep the hemoglobin level >10g/dl and to suppress the HbS level to <30% of the circulating red cells. A proliferative retinopathy requires opthalmological assessment with laser therapy to prevent bleeding.

In addition to SS disease, obstetricians must be aware of HbSC disease, where there may be essentially normal levels of hemoglobin during the pregnancy, such

Table 9.13 – Management of sickle-cell disorders in pregnancy

Diagnosis	Sickle test +ve, HbS and HbF present, but no HbA Sickle cells on blood film
Infection management	Penicillin Pneumovax Prompt recognition of respiratory tract infection (RTI)/ urinary tract infection (UTI) Malarial prophylaxis (if appropriate)
Pain management	Multidisciplinary action Controlled analgesia Day unit attendance
Renal management	Adequate hydration and urinary output Prompt infection treatment

Anemia management	Folate supplementation
	Iron supplements (if appropriate)
	Minimize red blood cell (rbc) alloimmunization
	Consider transfusion (reduce sickle-cells to <30%) in:
	    Pre-eclampsia (PET)
	    Preoperative work-up
	    Acute anemia
	    Septicemia
	    Acute renal failure
	    Acute chest syndrome
	    Recent cerebral ischemia of arterial origin (CIAO)
	    Multiple pregnancy

Delivery management	Planning, especially if placental insufficiency or poor maternal reserve
Neonatal screening	Counseling
Remember	Gallstone/cholecystitis risk Retinopathy risk

that the obstetrician and the mother are unaware of the problem. These women are, however, at risk of severe sickling crises during pregnancy and the peurperium.

Pregnancy-specific management

At the first antenatal visit the presence of any factors which could affect pregnancy outcome should be assessed. This includes the past obstetric history, evidence of chronic organ damage and the use of, and need for, narcotic analgesia. At all stages a multidisciplinary approach involving obstetrician, hematologist, anesthetist and general/infectious disease physician is required for appropriate management and planning of pregnancy cases.

The mainstays of management of a pregnancy in subjects with a severe sickling disorder are: folic acid supplementation (at a dose of at least 5mg/day for the whole pregnancy); regular hemoglobin level estimations; regular monitoring of fetal growth; consideration of regular transfusion when there is a twin or triplet pregnancy (see Table 9.13). The mother should be advised on the importance of the early recognition and treatment of infection, and the importance of maintaining adequate hydration. Screening for HIV, and hepatitis A, B and C should be carried out after suitable counseling. Routine urinalysis may assist in the detection of infection. As with other higher risk pregnancies, there should be regular monitoring of blood pressure and fetal development.

Randomized studies have shown no overall benefit in prophylactic blood transfusions in pregnant women, although there may be a reduction in the frequency of vaso-occlusive events when prophylactic transfusion has been used. Transfusion should be considered, however, when there is an acute anemia (hemoglobin level<5g/dl), pre-eclampsia, septicemia, acute renal failure, acute chest syndrome, a recent episode of CIAO and when preparing for surgery. As noted above, multiple pregnancy will require assessment for transfusion on a more regular basis, with the aim of maintaining HbS at <30% of circulating hemoglobin.

The management of an acute sickle-cell crisis in pregnancy should include hydration with intravenous fluids, pain control and the treatment of any associated infection. Both the mother and fetus may require oxygen therapy and the cardiotocography (CTG) may be non-reactive during a maternal crisis.

The timing of transfusion and the timing of delivery may be important factors in limiting maternal and fetal mortality, especially if there is evidence of placental insufficiency, or if there is a limitation of maternal cardiac, renal or hepatic reserve. Given the loss of fluids during delivery, close attention should be provided to maternal hydration, adequate pain control and oxygenation. After delivery, early mobilization and risk assessment for venous thrombosis and graduated elastic compression stockings and low-molecular-weight heparin (LMWH), should be used to prevent venous thromboembolism (VTE).

Although hydroxycarbamide (hydroxyurea) may ameliorate symptoms, by elevation of HbF levels and reduction of sickling episodes, it crosses the placenta and may have a teratogenic effect on the human fetus. In animal studies it has been associated with defects in the central nervous system, palate and skeleton, as well as cardiovascular and ocular abnormalities. It is also possible that it may induce myelosuppression in the fetus in the second and third trimesters. At present there is little information on the safety of this drug when those maintained on it prior to pregnancy conceive, although a number of normal pregnancy outcomes have been reported. However, as there is no evidence that it is beneficial to the mother or the fetus, as with the myeloproliferative disorders, it is probably best avoided, especially in the first trimester.

The principles of anesthesia in pregnant patients with major sickling disorders is similar to non-pregnant subjects, with the need to avoid dehydration and hypothermia, and fluid replacement should be supplied through a fluid warmer.

Regional anesthesia, both spinal and epidural, appear safe for operative and non-operative delivery, although epidural is often preferred. There must be, however, adequate hydration to avoid any hypotension occurring secondary to sympathetic blockade, but such blockade could, in theory, increase blood flow and reduce the risk of vaso-occlusion. As noted above, there is a need to consider thrombo-prophylaxis against VTE in such patients.

After delivery, there is a need to carefully attend to pain relief and hydration to counteract the effects of increased metabolism and diuresis, and so avoid sickling. In such circumstances, an acute chest crisis may be misdiagnosed as infection, fluid overload or a reaction to anesthesia.

Despite the improvements in feto-maternal outcomes in recent decades, mothers with a major sickling disorder are still at risk of renal, cardiovascular and cerebrovascular complications during pregnancy. In poorly developed countries a number of factors are important in the success of pregnancies. These include: adequate maternal nutrition; education on the nature of sickle-cell disorders; the early recognition and treatment of urinary and respiratory infections; the maintenance of adequate hydration and urinary output; the regular use of antimalarial prophylaxis; systematic supplementation with multivitamins, including folate and iron (depending on iron status); and the use of transfusion when the symptoms of anemia are intolerable or appear likely to lead to cardiac failure. In these populations, methods such as these may reduce the maternal and fetal mortality to a level comparable with local non-sickle-cell patients and with sickle patients in developed countries.

Other hemoglobinopathies

The combination of sickle-cell with HbC (HbSC) results in a lesser sickling disorder, although it carries a higher risk of retinopathy. The diagnosis can be suspected by the presence of a large number of target cells and sickle cells on the blood film and the presence of HbC on electrophoresis. However, both HbC and HbE disease (without S) are associated with a relatively mild anemia and splenomegaly, and often no specific treatment is required. Indeed, aside from mild anemia, which may be exacerbated by iron or folic acid deficiency, both HbCC and C/β^0 syndromes are likely to be associated with a normal pregnancy outcome.

Another Hb variant is HbD, which migrates to the same position as HbS on gel electrophoresis. In homozygous DD there is a mild hemolytic anemia, and when it occurs as a compound heterozygote with HbS it can result in a sickling disorder.

Heinz body anemias

A small deletion, or amino acid substitution, in the globin gene, affecting the protein structure of the globin molecule around the heme pocket, can result in a number of consequences. These include:

- Instability of the hemoglobin; or
- Easier oxidation of the heme moiety; or
- Hemoglobin precipitation (with the formation of so-called Heinz bodies within the red cell); or
- An altered oxygen affinity of the hemoglobin.

These disorders are associated with a lifelong tendency to hemolysis, which is exacerbated by infection or exposure to oxidative substances. The diagnosis can be made by finding a combination of hemolysis, hemoglobin instability on exposure to heat or isopropanol, exclusion of a more common hemoglobinopathy, and, in some cases, alteration in the oxygen dissociation (affinity) of the hemoglobin molecule.

Such mutations are not always associated with an abnormal electrophoretic pattern and may not always be associated with a family history. When such mutations increase the oxygen affinity, they may come to light in the investigation of erythrocytosis, and when they reduce the oxygen affinity they may result in the investigation of congenital cyanosis. There is little information on their impact in pregnancy.

Red cell membrane defects and enzymopathies

A variety of disorders of the red cell membrane or intracellular red cell enzymes may result in congenital hemolysis. The majority, such as hereditary spherocytosis, most often result in a mild hemolytic disorder which comes to light in childhood during an infection. When severe, these disorders are treated by splenectomy. As they are associated with chronic hemolysis, pregnant mothers are at increased risk of folic acid deficiency, leg ulcers and gallstones.

There are also a number of disorders of the red cell enzyme pathways which can result in:

- A reduction in adenosine triphosphate (ATP: a principal energy source for the cell); or
- A reduction in the reducing agents NADH or NADPH (the major antioxidant potential of the red cell); or
- A reduction in available 2,3-DPG, which may alter the hemoglobin's oxygen affinity.

A deficiency in the reducing agents NADH and NADPH will result in red cells which are at increased risk of hemolysis under oxidative stress. The commonest cause of this is a deficiency of the enzyme, glucose-6-phosphate dehydrogenase deficiency (G6PDH). The gene coding for G6PDH is found on the X chromosome, and although most common in the tropics, it is found in many other areas. The deficiency results in a lifelong tendency to hemolysis, often triggered by oxidative foods (classically the fava bean) and oxidative drugs (such as antimalarials and some vitamin K derivatives). Although it most often affects male carriers, it can also affect female carriers if there is excessive lyonization in the normal gene (see Chapter 4). Patients are most often well between the episodes of severe hemolysis. G6PDH deficiency is also associated with neonatal jaundice in an affected male. The mechanism for this is unclear, but the management is similar to other causes of neonatal jaundice, and includes phototherapy and, where necessary, exchange transfusion. There are a variety of methods for detection of G6PDH levels in the red cell that can be used to distinguish this disorder from other forms of Heinz-body-forming hemolysis.

The porphyrias

The porphyrias result from a number of inherited defects in the enzymes which are required for the synthesis of heme. Although there are a wide variety of molecular defects, seven clinical types of porphyria can be distinguished. These can be considered by whether the defect results in the accumulation of porphyrins (whose fluorescent properties result in the generation of free radicals and a marked, often scarring, photosensitive skin rash), porphyrin precursors (which result in neurological manifestations), or both. In some instances, the enzyme defects are inducible, which can lead to an acute disorder. The exact diagnosis is determined by the combination of detectable porphyrins and precursors in plasma, erythrocytes, urine and stool. The effect on hemoglobin production may be slight, as many of implicated enzymes are not rate limiting in heme biosynthesis, although there may be a mild hemolytic anemia.

Table 9.14 – Porphyria in pregnancy

Porphyria cutanea tarda (PCT)	First trimester has highest risk of symptoms
	There may be glucose intolerance
	There may be associated hepatitis C or B
	Avoid alcohol
	Avoid sun
	No routine iron
	If symptoms, venesect
	If refractory symptoms, consider chloroquine
Acute intermittent porphyria (AIP)	Avoid drugs/precipitants
	If symptoms:
	Remove precipitant
	Hydrate patient
	Carbohydrate supplements
	Hematin
	Pain control
	Seizure treatment

Of the seven types, congenital erythropoietic porphyria (CEP), porphyria cutanea tarda (PCT), erythropoietic protoporphyria (EPP) and acute intermittent porphyria (AIP) have been reported to be influenced by pregnancy, or to affect pregnancy management (Table 9.14) The prevalence in European populations is estimated at around 1 in 1 000 000 for CEP, 1 in 25 000–70 000 for PCT, 1 in 75 000–200 000 for EPP and 1–2 in 100 000 for clinically overt AIP. The actual prevalence of AIP is, however, likely to be around 10 times higher, as 90% of subjects have latent disease. Although a number of 'bedside' tests are available for porphyrias, their investigation is best carried out in a center with expertise in this area.

CEP

In CEP there is often severe, cutaneous, scarring, photosensitivity that is evident from childhood. This is accompanied by a normochromic, normocytic anemia, with basophilic stippling evident in the red cell and nucleated erythrocytes a common feature.

Standard suncreams are often ineffective, as they do not screen out the wavelengths of around 400nm that lead to the photosensitivity. Reflective creams, with zinc or titanium, may be effective. Other strategies such as activated charcoal (binding bile porphyrin) and hypertransfusion (to suppress endogenous erythropoiesis) have been used successfully in some cases. If anemia is a problem, it may respond to splenectomy.

One of the CEP mutations is associated with severe disease, which can result in non-immune hydrops fetalis, or transfusion-dependant anemia from birth. In many cases, prenatal diagnosis from amniotic cells is possible.

PCT

PCT results from a reduction in activity of one of the heme synthesis enzymes in the liver. This leads to an accumulation of uropophyrins in the plasma, which are excreted in the urine. PCT results in marked skin fragility in light-exposed areas, facial hypertrichosis and hyperpigmentation. It is not, however, associated with neuropsychiatric disturbance. It presents late, often in association with alcohol excess, iron overload and/or hepatitis B or C carriage.

Exogenous estrogen is associated with expression of PCT and it has also been diagnosed for the first time in pregnancy, although there is debate as to whether pregnancy exacerbates the disease or not. If exacerbation does occur, this is likely to be in the first trimester, as there is a reduction in urine porphyrin and placenta-derived estrogen and progestogen production in the second trimester.

In pregnancy, it would be sensible to monitor known cases (as there may be a greater risk of glucose intolerance), to minimize exposure to alcohol and sunlight, and to refrain from iron supplementation. In non-pregnant subjects, avoidance of alcohol, removal of iron by venesection, recombinant erythopoietin and treatment of hepatitis C, if present, with α-interferon have all been reported as beneficial. In symptomatic and refractory cases in pregnancy, venesection and chloroquine have both been used, although chloroquine is known to be teratogenic in animals.

EPP

EPP results from a defect in ferrochelatase, which is the last enzyme in the heme pathway. The level of the enzyme does not, however, correlate well with symptoms. EPP most often becomes evident in childhood, with exposure to sunlight leading to itching and burning, and local erythema. It can also present in the differential diagnosis of a sideroblastic anemia and, in later life, may lead to gallstones due to precipitated protoporphyrin. Rarely, it may manifest with a neurological crisis resembling AIP.

EPP is diagnosed by the detection of elevated levels of erythrocyte-derived free protophorphyrin. Although elevated levels also occur in iron deficiency and lead poisoning, the levels in EPP are usually considerably higher than those in iron deficiency (normal <50µg/dl, iron deficiency anemia (IDA) <300µg/dl, EPP and lead poisoning 300–4500µg/dl), but unlike lead poisoning and iron deficiency, the protophorphyrin of EPP is non-chelated.

Treatments include avoidance of sun exposure, zinc- or titanium-based sunscreens, induction of hypercarotenemia (which can reduce photosensitivity), hematin therapy (which reduces the production of porphyrins and their precursors), cholestyramine (which binds bile protoporphyrins) and activated charcoal. It is possible that there may be an improvement in symptoms in pregnancy, although this requires confirmation and the mechanism of such an improvement is unknown.

AIP

AIP results from a decreased conversion of porphobilinogen to prophyrins. It is transmitted as an autosomal dominant condition, with the majority of cases due to single base mutations. The mechanism of neurotoxicity is unknown, but could be due to a rise in the porphyrin precursor 5-aminolevulinic acid (which may inhibit neurotransmitters), or a depletion of cellular heme (leading to reduction in energy production in neural tissues).

The condition is characterized by the acute onset of autonomic neuropathy, which commonly presents with abdominal pain, constipation, tachycardia, hypertension and vomiting. This may be accompanied by acute anxiety, confusion, psychosis and seizures. In 50% of subjects, persisting hypertension and renal impairment may also occur. The blood count is usually normal aside from a raised white cell count in the acute phase. Both 5-aminolevulinic acid and porphobilinogen can be detected in the urine, especially during an acute attack.

A number of circumstances can lead to an acute attack. These include gonadal hormones (particularly progestogens), decreased caloric intake, alcohol and other drugs (usually by induction of cytochrome p450 leading to an increased need for intracellular heme), such as barbiturates, valproate, nifedipine and diclofenac. It is impossible to predict whether a drug will or will not produce a reaction, but drugs such as opiates, corticosteroids, vitamin C, aspirin, insulin, nitrous oxide and labetolol are generally considered to be safe. A fuller list of drugs thought to be suitable or unsuitable is to be found in the British National Formulary (www.bnf.org).

The management of an acute event requires removal of any precipitating factors, appropriate hydration and carbohydrate supplementation (by nasogastric feeding). If attacks do not improve within 24 hours, therapy with intravenous hematin has been suggested. The dose is of the order of 3mg/kg, once daily, for 4 days. As too rapid an infusion may cause irritation at the injection site, it should be given through central venous access. In addition, too high a dose may result in renal failure. After treatment, the symptoms of AIP usually improve within 48 hours. The treatment of seizures can be problematic, as many antiepileptic medications are also associated with AIP. Possible options include correction of any hyponatremia and treatment with clonazepam or magnesium sulfate.

Reports of AIP in pregnancy are not common, with an attack rate, in those known to have porphyria, of 16% in the antenatal and 8% in the postnatal period. Although estrogen is capable of inducing heme synthesis, other features of pregnancy, such as hyperemesis (leading to calorie loss) or metoclopramide therapy, may precipitate an attack. Initial reports suggested a dire outcome for those with AIP, but more recent work suggests that, with adequate maternal care, a good outcome is possible. A recent study has suggested that miscarriage may be more common in symptomatic AIP patients when compared with those with latent disease, but this observation requires confirmation. In this study, around 20% of subjects reported an improvement, around 10% a decline and around 70% no change in symptoms during pregnancy. The risk of an acute episode, however, cannot be predicted in a primigravid subject, and AIP may be confused with symptoms of hyperemesis, eclampsia and even (when there is a progressive muscle weakness) Guillain-Barré syndrome in pregnancy.

The management of an acute episode in pregnancy follows the same principles outlined above. Although caution is recommended with hematin (haem arginate) in pregnancy, it has been used with success in pregnant subjects. When the diagnosis is made for the first time, it should be remembered that other family members should be screened for the disorder.

Index